CULTURE AND RETARDATION

CULTURE, ILLNESS, AND HEALING

CULTURE AND RETARDATION

Life Histories of Mildly Mentally Retarded Persons in American Society

Edited by

L. L. LANGNESS

*Departments of Psychiatry and Anthropology, University of California,
Los Angeles, California, U.S.A.*

and

HAROLD G. LEVINE

*Graduate School of Education, University of California,
Los Angeles, California, U.S.A.*

D. REIDEL PUBLISHING COMPANY

A MEMBER OF THE KLUWER 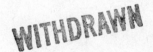 ACADEMIC PUBLISHERS GROUP

DORDRECHT / BOSTON / LANCASTER / TOKYO

Library of Congress Cataloging-in-Publication Data

Culture and retardation

   (Culture, illness, and healing)
   Bibliography: p.
   Includes index.
   1. Mentally handicapped – United States – Biography. 2. Cognition and culture – United States. 3. Stigma (Social psychology) I. Langness, L. L. (Lewis L.), 1929– . II. Levine, Harold Gary, 1945– . III. Series.
   HV3006.A38C85   1986   362.3′092′2 [B]   86–13735
   ISBN 90–277–2177–7

Published by D. Reidel Publishing Company,
P.O. Box 17, 3300 AA Dordrecht, Holland.

Sold and distributed in the U.S.A. and Canada
by Kluwer Academic Publishers,
101 Philip Drive, Assinippi Park, Norwell, MA 02061, U.S.A.

In all other countries, sold and distributed
by Kluwer Academic Publishers Group,
P.O. Box 322, 3300 AH Dordrecht, Holland.

TABLE OF CONTENTS

INTRODUCTION

Mental retardation in the United States is currently defined as ". . . signif-icantly subaverage general intellectual functioning existing concurrently with deficits in adaptive behavior, and manifested during the development period" (Grossman, 1977). Of the estimated six million plus mentally retarded individuals in this country fully 75 to 85% are considered to be "func-tionally" retarded (Edgerton, 1984). That is, they are mildly retarded persons with no evident organic etiology or demonstrable brain pathology.

Despite the relatively recent addition of adaptive behavior as a factor in the definition of retardation, I.Q. still remains as the essential diagnostic criterion (Edgerton, 1984: 26). An I.Q. below 70 indicates subaverage functioning. However, even such an "objective" measure as I.Q. is prob-lematic since a variety of data indicate quite clearly that cultural and social factors are at play in decisions about who is to be considered "retarded" (Edgerton, 1968; Kamin, 1974; Langness, 1982).

Thus, it has been known for quite some time that there is a close relationship between socio-economic status and the prevalence of mild mental retardation: higher socio-economic groups have fewer mildly retarded persons than lower groups (Hurley, 1969). Similarly, it is clear that ethnic minorities in the United States — Blacks, Mexican-Americans, American Indians, Puerto Ricans, Hawaiians, and others — are disproportionately represented in the retarded population (Mercer, 1968; Ramey *et al.*, 1978). At a more global level some have argued that mentally retarded persons are merely a "surplus" population in a society that is unwilling to provide them with jobs or otherwise care for them (Farber, 1968; Scull, 1978). This is a surplus, moreover, that can be easily increased or decreased by moving the I.Q. cut-off score a few points in the requisite direction.

That the relationship between I.Q. and mental retardation is problematic is further borne out by the report of the President's Committee on Mental Retardation, *The Six-Hour Retarded Child* (1970): "We now have what may be called a 6-hour retarded child — retarded from 9 to 3, five days a week, solely on the basis of an I.Q. score, without regard to his adaptive behavior, which may be exceptionally adaptive to the situation and community in which he lives" (1970: frontispiece). It is also known that many supposedly retarded persons simply disappear into the wider community when they leave school and as they become older. What is not known is why some do and others do not, and how this process of disappearance and adaptation actually works, problems that lend themselves to ethnographic methods since they cannot be understood through the use of questionnaires or other short-term research techniques (Edgerton, 1984).

L. L. Langness and H. G. Levine (eds.), Culture and Retardation, ix—xv.
© *1986 by D. Reidel Publishing Company.*

In spite of the role of culture in the definition and nature of mental retardation, as late as 1968 both Kirk (1968: v) and Edgerton (1968) remarked on the paucity of sociological and anthropological research in this area, and the late Harvey Dingman published "A Plea for Social Research in Mental Retardation" (1968). Edgerton stated the situation very clearly at that time:

When the various versions of social science were staking their claims to certain aspects of the study of man's doings, mental retardation remained a *tertium quid* — not quite within the domain of any social discipline. And so, rejected by the sciences of what is social and cultural, mental retardation has continued to be seen as a problem for physicians, psychologists or educators. That mental retardation should not have been viewed as grist for the theoretical mill of sociology or anthropology is particularly odd, because mental illness has long been regarded by sociologists and anthropologists alike as a particularly fruitful source of insights concerning the nature of man-in-society. There are many reasons why mental illness has become a properly accredited area of study in social science, while mental retardation has not, but most of these reasons need not concern us here. What should concern us is the mystifying fact that so many social scientists (and here anthropologists are more guilty than sociologists) do not regard mental retardation as a social or cultural phenomenon. I say mystifying, because nothing in the probabilistic world of social scientific reality is more certain than the assertion that mental retardation is a socio-cultural problem through and through (1968: 75—76).

Mercer has stated that her review of etiological studies abstracted in *Mental Retardation Abstracts* for the period 1964—1967 revealed that only 0.1% of the 2013 studies dealt with "functional" as contrasted with "organic" retardation (1973: 11). Such studies focused exclusively on biological as opposed to sociocultural factors. Research dealing specifically with the social and cultural factors relating to mental retardation has accelerated somewhat in recent years, but this is still limited in scope, amount, and location (Edgerton, 1984).

Edgerton's pioneering work, *The Cloak of Competence* (1967), set the stage for the more anthropological, naturalistic, longitudinal and qualitative research that has become a tradition at the UCLA Mental Retardation Research Center. The Socio-behavioral Group, which Edgerton was instrumental in assembling, consists of anthropologists, linguists, psychologists and educators. The research conducted by this group has centered on the lives of mentally retarded adults after they have left school. It has attempted to follow them as they react and adapt (or fail to adapt) to the demands of everyday life. Concentrating on those retarded individuals with the best chance of living independently or "disappearing" into the community, the UCLA researchers have monitored the lives of a large sample of clients with I.Q.'s in the 60s and low 70s and with no formal record of physical, speech, or psychiatric impairment.

One fundamental finding about mildly retarded persons living in the community is that, "in general, their lives are complex, partly concealed from investigation and highly changeable" (Edgerton, 1984: 32). This implies, among other things, that those who wish to understand the lives of such people would do well to be patient and must be willing to spend a great deal of time with them. Indeed, Edgerton believes it requires a minimum of one year of intensive ethnographic research before even accurate baseline data can be assured (1984: 32). Edgerton continues: "The majority are anything but stable. Their lives often change abruptly, dramatically and unpredictably. Crises of all sorts occur in their lives . . . but mentally retarded persons seldom have resources that can quickly stabilize their lives. Agencies are slow to react, supporters are unreliable, and credit cards, bank accounts, insurance policies and union memberships are typically absent altogether" (1984: 33).

In any thoroughgoing ethnographic study of mentally retarded individuals, anthropologists must be sensitive to the beliefs and values that parents, social workers, doctors, and just plain citizens bring to their experience of and with the retarded. Perhaps the best single reason for this is the idea held by many Americans, in all walks of life, that the mentally retarded and others who are "different" are "like children". This idea is clearly part of our own cultural heritage, dating at least to the Greeks who drew an analogy between the infancy of the child and the infancy of civilization, and was formalized during the 19th century when it became an integral part of evolutionary theory as applied to society and culture. In this theory children were equated with "savages", and contemporary "primitive" peoples with our prehistoric ancestors. The theory also tended to associate childlike thought and behavior with women, the mentally ill, criminals, and others (Langness, 1985).

The effects of this belief that equates retarded behavior with child behavior on the lives of the retarded cannot be overestimated. It is this belief that enables us to consider retarded persons, even adults, to be irresponsible and to treat them accordingly. It allows us to categorize them as incompetent and thus to overlook whatever competencies they may have or might well learn if taught properly. It enables us to assume they inevitably have bad judgment, do not know what they want, and cannot be trusted. It allows us on the one hand to overprotect them and on the other to ignore them. It is not unusual in this context, for example, to see doctors refuse to speak directly to an adult retarded patient but address their comments instead to the parent standing next to them. While the mildly retarded have their problems, to be sure, it is clear to those who have worked closely with them over long periods of time and on a day-to-day basis that the beliefs and attitudes predicated on the cultural assumption that they are childlike are vastly oversimplified and certainly harmful with respect to their potential "normalization" or independent living.

The papers that make up this volume are the result of an ethnographic approach and offer a somewhat more detailed view of the lives of the retarded than is ordinarily achieved. Although they represent only a small fraction of the total population we have worked with over the years, the points they make are more broadly applicable to this wider population. In the concluding chapter we try to outline in what ways this is so.

The methods employed by the UCLA team of researchers have been described in detail elsewhere (Edgerton and Langness, 1978). They consist primarily of long-term naturalistic observations in multiple settings, participant-observation, and life histories. They emphasize rapport, detail, multiple points of view, and, above all, context. As the life history method features so prominently in our research, the first paper reviews the biographical materials available on mentally retarded persons and attempts to explain the benefits that can be derived from the application of life history taking to such a population. In so doing it also places the papers that follow in historical and intellectual perspective. Although none of the papers offers a complete, or even near complete, life history, all of them have been written with an eye to the overall historical, social, familial, and cultural context in which the subject of the study finds him or herself immersed. They could as easily be called case studies although we feel they offer more context and detail than what we ordinarily conceive of as case studies. These are the kinds of papers, we note, that find their way to publication only with great difficulty. This is in large part because the available outlets for mental retardation research are geared almost exclusively towards formulaic, virtually ritualized quantification, and also tend to impose prohibitive page limitations. This situation is, of course, an obvious cultural artifact, part of the scientism that has arisen out of the attempt by social scientists to be "truly scientific". The reader must judge for him or herself whether or not the present collection contributes to an understanding of the phenomenon of mental retardation.

Naturally there are many problems and pitfalls in attempting detailed life or case histories with the retarded. Korbin's paper illustrates this very well. Working with a child, and with a Down syndrome child at that, she found it virtually impossible to construct a satisfactory account. Life histories of children and the retarded (especially the more seriously retarded) have seldom been attempted not only because of the difficulty, but also because of the expectation of researchers that children and the retarded are either unable to recount anything of their lives or their lives are so uninteresting as to be a waste of time. It is clear that even Sarah has skills that are unexpected, and doubtless she has much more potential than has ever been realized; yet the problems of communication, interviewing, and observation are apparent.[1] We include Korbin's paper here not only as an example of these problems, but also because it makes an extremely important point that recurs more implicitly in many of the other papers: the lives of mentally retarded persons seem to get increasingly out of synchronization with what might be regarded as the "normal" life course. This comes about as a result of natural maturation and aging in conflict with cultural expectations about the "normal" course of development. It is also, we believe, a result of faulty and incomplete socialization, a point we discuss at greater length in the concluding chapter.

Kaufman's essay shows how, by attempting to step back from her personal involvement with her "subject" and employing social science methods, she was able to come to a greater understanding of her handicapped daughter. It also illustrates how one's attitudes and values shape expectations, in this case expectations that changed rather dramatically as she began to see her daughter's life in a more complete context. Paradoxically, her daughter came to change her own values so that they more closely approximated those of her mother's. In a modest way this is perhaps an example of how an "outsider" comes to grasp an "insider's" point of view.

The paper on Larry B. follows the life of a retarded individual over a six year period as he moves from a board and care facility through a number of classes and training programs which prepare him to live independently in his own apartment. It documents his attempts to deal with this experience and with the frustrations of both board and care life and of living independently.

Tim Anthony is a remarkable case of an individual who, by all ordinary expectations, should have turned out to be a genuine problem child with a virtually hopeless prognosis for living a decent life. Yet, somehow, he manages to overcome his traumatic childhood and develops aspirations which, while he will have great difficulty in achieving them, nonetheless motivate him to keep going and try to constantly improve himself.

Koegel's first paper deals with the socialization of handicapped individuals and how, even with the best of intentions, they are treated differently from "normals". Koegel argues that retarded persons are socialized for incompetence; and he explores the process by which faulty socialization can build on itself in such a way that it is virtually impossible for a person once labeled retarded to cope adequately with his or her social and material environment.

Edgerton's paper carries Koegel's argument one step further by demonstrating the virtual impossibility of living a "normal" life after being "delabeled". And delabeling, as he points out, is a far more common phenomenon in the lives of retarded individuals than one might expect. Once one has lived as retarded, been systematically denied information about the everyday world, provided with false information, his or her chances for subsequent normal development are slim. Both Edgerton's and Koegel's papers suggest the critical importance of studies of adult socialization among the handicapped, an issue raised in the 1960s for non-handicapped adults (Brim and Wheeler, 1966), but in research vogue only in the last ten years.

Koegel's second paper, focusing on the social support for a retarded adult, perhaps comes closer to being a life history. Certainly it is a relatively detailed account of a life style that, while it may seem offensive to some, seems to be a successful adaption to life's demands for the woman involved. Through the use of this abbreviated life history Koegel makes clear the shifting and unpredictable nature of social support systems but also the importance of having a predictable income. Indeed, in spite of Koegel's optimistic speculation on Penny's ability to get by, it would appear that without her financial support her life would be even more unpredictable and almost certainly more unpleasant.

The final paper by Whittemore deals with the life of Ted Barrett, a man the Socio-Behavioral group has followed for more than 20 years. Here is a life presented genuinely in context, with all the complexities of coping, maneuvering, and negotiating that inform the day-to-day lives of the mildly retarded living in the broader community. Whatever else it does, Mr. Barrett's story illustrates that the handicapped are not without ability and that they can and do confront their problems with a variety of solutions which, although they might not always seem the "right" ones to us, do "make sense" given the idiosyncrasies of one person's life.

Before the reader goes on to the individual life stories presented here we wish to introduce one significant caveat. While very few people still seriously or unthinkingly believe that intelligence or adaptation to life can be reduced to simple, unidimensional numerical scores or that scientific understanding is furthered only through tightly controlled experimental studies, those who remain intransigent in their beliefs will doubtless find numerous objections to the studies and point of view to be found here. Our primary reasons for putting this book together were precisely to show that mentally retarded persons are enormously complex in their personalities, behavior, and abilities, that failure in one set of (I.Q.) tests for such persons does not necessarily mean failure in other areas of their lives, and that retarded persons are anything but a single homogeneous group best characterized as an I.Q. range. Sadly, acknowledgement of these insights has been late in coming. With this collection of papers we hope to further encourage an emerging new view of retarded individuals, one in which their essential humanity is not ignored in favor of economics and efficiency and one in which the true complexity of their lives can be fully appreciated and subjected to study.

NOTE

1. That is it not impossible to do fairly sophisticated life history work even with Down's individuals see Kristina Kennann's recent *Time in Her Life: A Down's Woman's Personal Account* (1984) in which she discusses this in detail and gives a fascinating account of how one such individual uses her idiosyncratic sense of time to organize her life and maintain her interpersonal relations.

REFERENCES

Brim, O. and Wheeler, S.
   1966 *Socialization after childhood: Two essays.* New York: John Wiley and Sons.
Dingman, H. F.
   1968 A plea for social research in mental retardation. *American Journal of Mental Deficiency,* 73(1): 2—4.
Edgerton, R. B.
   1967 *The cloak of competence: Stigma in the lives of the mentally retarded.* Berkeley: University of California Press.

Edgerton, R. B.
1968 Anthropology and mental retardation: A plea for the comparative study of incompetence. *In* H. J. Prem, L. A. Hammerlynck and J. E. Crosson (eds.), *Behavioral research in mental retardation*. Rehabilitation Research and Training Center in Mental Retardation, University of Oregon, Eugene.
Edgerton, R. B.
1984 Anthropology and mental retardation: Research approaches and opportunities. *Culture, Medicine, and Psychiatry, 8*: 25—48.
Edgerton, R. B. and Langness, L. L.
1978 Observing mentally retarded persons in community settings: An anthropological perspective. *In* G. P. Sackett (ed.), *Observing behavior, Vol. 1*. Baltimore: University Park Press.
Farber, B.
1968 *Mental retardation: Its social context and social consequences*. Boston: Houghton Mifflin Co.
Grossman, H. J.
1977 *A manual on terminology and classification in mental retardation*. Washington, D. C.: American Association on Mental Deficiency, Special Publication No. 2.
Hurley, R. L.
1969 *Poverty and mental retardation: A causal relationship*. New York: Vintage Press.
Kamin, L. J.
1974 *The science and politics of I. Q.* Potomac, Maryland: Erlbaum.
Kirk, S. A.
1968 Introduction. *In* Bernard Farber, *Mental retardation: Its social context and social consequences*. Boston: Houghton-Mifflin.
Langness, L. L.
1982 Mental retardation as an anthropological problem. Wenner-Gren Foundation Working Papers in the Anthropology of the Handicapped No. 1.
Langness, L. L.
1986 *The study of culture* (revised edition). Novato, California: Chandler and Sharp.
Mercer. J. R.
1968 Sociological perspectives on mild mental retardation. *In* H. C. Haywood (ed.), *Socio-cultural aspects of mental retardation* (pp. 378—391). New York: Appleton-Century Crofts.
Mercer. J. R.
1973 *Labeling the mentally retarded: Clinical and social system perspectives on mental retardation*. Berkeley and Los Angeles: University of California Press.
President's Committee on Mental Retardation.
1970 The six-hour retarded child: A report on a conference on problems of education of children in the inner-city. Washington, D. C.: U.S. Government Printing Office.
Ramey, C. T., Stedman, D. J., Borders-Patterson, A. and Megel, W.
1978 Predicting school failure from information available at brith. *American Journal of Mental Deficiency, 82*: 525—534.
Scull, A. T.
1977 *Community treatment and the deviant — A radical view*. Englewood Cliffs, New Jersey: Prentice Hall.

L. L. LANGNESS   HAROLD G. LEVINE
Depts. of Psychiatry and Anthropology,   *Graduate School of Education,*
University of California,   *University of California,*
Los Angeles   *Los Angeles*

ROBERT D. WHITTEMORE, L. L. LANGNESS, PAUL KOEGEL

THE LIFE HISTORY APPROACH TO MENTAL RETARDATION

Anthropologists, in their attempt to understand the multiple life ways of human beings, have long insisted on having an emic, or insider's point of view. Bronislaw Malinowski, whose methods were the precursor of anthropological fieldwork as now practiced, emphasized that the ethnographer's final goal is "to grasp the native's point of view, his relation to life, to realize *his* vision of *his* world" (1922: 25). As anthropologists who have turned our attention to the study of the mentally retarded, we attempt to remain faithful to this point of view. One of the methods we employ for this purpose is the taking of life histories.

Life histories have long been a kind of common denominator for the social, behavioral, and medical sciences (Langness, 1964; Frank, 1979; Langness and Frank, 1981). This biographical approach is employed by historians, folklorists, and others in the humanities. It is also a well-established literary genre, one written and enjoyed by professionals and nonprofessionals alike. Quite a number of people, mostly nonprofessionals, have written biographical and quasi-biographical accounts of their experiences with mental retardation. In this paper, we wish to review these accounts, discuss our own approach, and consider the implications of our work for the understanding and treatment of the retarded.

LIFE HISTORIES OF THE MENTALLY RETARDED: AN OVERVIEW

In the materials reviewed[1], the lack of anything approximating an emic, or insider's view, is perhaps the most striking common feature. With very few exceptions (Bogdan and Taylor, 1976; Hunt, 1967; McCune, 1973; Seagoe, 1964; Turner, 1980), the literature is void of the experience it would presumably portray — that of the retarded individual, in his or her own voice. Nearly half of the 23 accounts of which we have taken note are brief sketches which portray some particular aspect of a retarded individual's being that has captured the observer's attention. Insights an author stresses in viewing the life of an institutionalized adult are often merely, as one author puts it "aspects of a man who might have been" (Cassel, 1948). Such a pointillistic interpretation of the life of the mentally retarded individual can lead the reader to conclude, just as some writers have concluded, that the life of a retarded man or woman is as simple as a "little song" (Nash, 1949) or, on the other hand, a complex spiritual burden to be borne by only the most dedicated of parents.

Longer non-clinical life accounts almost invariably tell, more than the

1

L. L. Langness and H. G. Levine (eds.), Culture and Retardation, 1—18.
© 1986 *by D. Reidel Publishing Company.*

story of the disabled person, the trials of the parent of guardian. Thus, beginning with Pearl Buck's (1950) moving retrospective of her child (who interestingly, remains nameless throughout her account) and continuing with such self-absorbed documents as J. Greenfield's *A Child Called Noah* (1965), we find a tradition which is rich not in the beliefs, perceptions, attitudes, feeling, or desires of the retarded, but with the problems and insights of parents as they adjust to their children's disabilities. It is as if the retarded do not have feelings or desires or life histories, or, if they do, they are somehow inconsequential.

The portrait of *non-retarded family* members which emerges from this literature reveals the extent to which such sources can contribute to our understanding of the impact a retarded individual has on his or her family. Expectant parents' anticipation of a child's promise turns to pain when an infant is identified as being handicapped. Early in the child's life, intense concern and anxiety over (a) physiognomy, particularly among mothers of Down's syndrome infants, and (b) developmental accomplishments are evident in the scrupulously detailed accounts of the motor and verbal control of the child. Optimism that friends' comments, and even professional diagnoses, could be mistaken fades as the disability becomes more visible and development increasingly violates what we think of as the normal chronology. Parental rebellion at the life prospects for themselves and their disabled offspring elicits prolonged and painful introspection. Self-recriminations regarding possibly mismanaged pregnancy, guilt over fantasizing the destruction or accidental death of the infant, are common. But such acute rejection of the self or offspring yields to concern over the child's potential impact on (a) siblings, (b) parental well-being, (c) the neighborhood into which the stigmatized child will be introduced, and (d) the stamina the family has to provide adequate care and an optimal growth environment for the disabled youth. If the handicapped child does not die in infancy, parental resolve to protect and occasionally, with assiduousness, to teach the child to read or write may build a certain "meaning out of meaninglessness" for the families involved. Subsequent familial reaction to a child's aggressive and destructive behavior and/or communicative difficulties may lead to alienation among family members. Parents can become isolated from their peers, normal siblings can become resentful of parental attention directed too exclusively to the handicapped member, and the family as a whole can become defensive and even fearful over the time and space devoted to the disabled child's needs and behavior.

During the course of these developmental changes in family orientation to the disabled child, oppressive curiosity and gratuitous advice from friends or relatives can be both disturbing and disruptive. Doctors, psychologists, and most others rarely support home residency or underscore the positive signs of a child's developmental progress. Extra-familial opinions, as professional advice or neighborhood concern, often incite enough parental doubt or community suspicion to tip the balance in favor of institutionalization. Depending upon both the particular bias of this advice and the nature and strength of the personal convictions of the parents, a disabled individual's right to life and happiness becomes the rationale either for or against institutionalization.

Usually, even for those who choose institutionalization, an effort is made to extract some meaningful lesson from having had a handicapped child as a family member. For families continuing to live in the disabled member's company, humility and tolerance may emerge. There is often a new acceptance of life and the problems of living, one which emphasizes the constructive importance of love and displays an increasing impatience with intolerance and misunderstanding. One disabled child lends her psychologist parent a new and vital perspective on brain damage and psychiatric disorders, another inspires parental commitment to world-wide research in retardation.

It is remarkable indeed, in light of the complete and variegated course traced by larger accounts of familial adjustment and adaptation, that the retarded individual exists mostly as a background influence and rarely as a receptive, rejecting, or contributing family member. Pearl Buck's (1950) portrayal of "those who know dimly that they are not as others are" must leave us uneasy because it is she alone who delineates this isolation from other human beings. Only suggestively in her portrayal of her daughter's clutched struggle with a pen's uncontrollability do we begin to suspect the pain the daughter herself feels as she strains to please mother, a friend, or some link outside herself. Here, and as a rule, the attempt is not to paint a portrait of the retarded family member as a feeling human being engaged in a personal struggle of his or her own. Rather, we see the rendering of the retarded as an assemblage of isolated character traits — as individuals with the love of music, the capacity for kindness, the desire to be liked, and so on. While we do see ample justification for parents to adduce, as does Murray (1956), that a retarded individual is "bewildered and confused . . . unable to cope with problems of ordinary existence", there is simply never enough data to provide the background to such a profile and consequently to assess what could be done to change it. These are not truly the stories of Barbara, Jan, Joey, Johnny, Virginia, Marc, Teddy, Eddie, Karen, Duncan, or David. Indeed, the ubiquitous tendency to use only first names in the titles of these works indicates to us that these are not meant to be truly biographies of the retarded but, rather, autobiographies of parents or siblings. Nigel Hunt, in *The World of Nigel Hunt* (1967), Billy McCune, in *The Autobiography of Billy McCune* (1973), are much more immediately recognizable as fully autonomous persons than those who exist for us only as first names, spoken about only by others, and thus, however, subconsciously, connoted as childlike or incompetent. While we realize that the goal of anonymity is often involved here, it seems to us that there may be a deeper explanation as well.

We have found only four works which represent truly autobiographical accounts by retarded persons: the diary of Nigel Hunt (1967), a compendium of diary notes by Paul Scott (Seagoe, 1964), and a narrative by Billy McCune (1973)[2] with a newspaper journalist's assistance and a recent Ph.D. dissertation in which a Downs woman collaborates in a life history (Kennann, 1984). Although the first two of these are editorialized, they must be seen as major contributions to a deepening sense of the retarded individual's self. Both are Down's individuals, and they both organize their accounts, as we all do, around events which were bits and pieces of their lives.

Nigel Hunt, almost as a master of ceremonies, guides the reader through his European tour experiences with his parents. On two occasions when he departs his parents' company, a self-assuredness and a competence emerge which may suggest that Hunt's description of these adventures as "being lost" may simply be borrowed from his parents. He is less forgetfully bewildered than temporarily and independently absorbed. It is clear that it was Hunt's parents' refusal to accept the advice of experts, those who were blind to a range of tasks which Hunt *could* perform, and their subsequent efforts to socialize him toward independence and competence, which instilled such exuberant initiative in their son. In Nigel Hunt's failure to indicate at any point that he felt stigmatized or thought of himself as handicapped, there is an essence of self-assured adaptiveness which says more about him as a human being than as an isolate. He appears neither as a "being apart" (Buck, 1950), nor as simply the personification of Down's "syndrome" which is what the forward to the work, written by neurologist Penrose, emphasizes.

Paul Scott (Seagoe, 1964), another Down's individual, initiates the first of many vanishing episodes at fourteen years of age. Again, the impression from Scott's diaries is that not once was he "lost" in the confused way his father and tutor-companion first thought him to be. Seagoe suggests that what psychologists later called "schizophrenic detachment" was not so much actually a running *from* a particular situation as it was *towards* one which Scott believed would be better. Such restlessness throughout Scott's life begins with his father's refusal to accept a private residential placement for his son, and, particularly after receiving private tutoring, grows in the context of thirteen years of travel with his father and tutor-companion.

In the course of these travels, Scott's increasing spontaneity of expression in diary entries, discrimination in tastes, his observational talents, personal involvement, projective concerns and imagination, his sense of personal pleasure and amusement, and imaginary fluency in pidgin Spanish all speak eloquently of a developing character profile. Scott, like Hunt, has very little to say in an introspective way about himself. But the contrasts in style and content he provides in his observations during his travels, as well as Seagoe's portrait of his residential period and more isolated later years, make a statement which is highly personal. Years of education and experience gave Scott, Seagoe believes, the tools to adapt to his eventual institutionalization. She comments, "He will trade spontaneity for conformity, avoid the demands he cannot accept, and escape through fantasy when he must . . . he will have his rich memories" (1964: 229).

Scott's account does suggest that a retarded individual him or herself can see in life an opportunity for formative growth, and "passages" (such as the trials of illness and aging) from which personal strength can be derived. Paul Scott prospers until, later in life, he faces the residential facility of which he never really becomes a part. Scott's lonely vigil of defiance and resistance, given the remarkable record of his youth, is much less an example of pathology than the final statement of a resolute attempt at adaptive competence. Neither Scott nor Hunt are the helpless, involuntary victims of genetic adversity, or the degenerated shells of individuals who "might have been".

For the experience of the *mildly* retarded, McCune's autobiography stands as a unique example of the type of work of which we wish to see more. McCune warns us not to "try to read between the lines, or to interpret this material as if it were a parable. Just interpret each word from your standard dictionary and I feel you will not go wrong" (1973: 31). He gives us a great deal, and the unsettling feeling of having to read between the lines as in other accounts is indeed relatively absent here.

Initially categorized "feebleminded" at sixteen, and then reclassified "normal" two years after, on the basis of I.Q. scores alone, McCune suffers a stormy enlistment in the Navy, is arrested and convicted as a rapist, publicly labeled a "sex criminal", and finally mutilates his sexual organs as a response to media sensationalism of his case. His personal sense of having been labeled and set apart from the stream of humanity is overwhelming. This being the case, there is a sense of isolation which other accounts of the marginal retarded individual only imply. In his account, he is the unwitting character, the flawed journeyman waiting to be snared. He says, "I became what I felt I had to in order to survive. I acted like the type of people I came in contact with" (1973: 28), and because of this he sees himself as having become a social problem: "I could not analyze my sense of what was right and wrong, nor the problems that I present to society . . . Perhaps I had a low-grade philosophical view of human existence . . . The philosophy of myself as a low-grade human being . . . Life is a race, and usually a long lonely one" (p. 28).

Nowhere is his isolation, his sense of self as a "low degree", more evident than in his description of others "just watching" him and of the mechanical quality to the interpersonal relations in his existence at the time of his unsought for yet seemingly fated meeting with Effie Leon in the back seat of her parked car. In his meeting with a court appointed psychiatrist, despite his fear of death in the electric chair and of incarceration in a mental institution, he is unable to manipulate the examination. "It is not what the individual human wants, but what the system needs. We are the garbage. They are the collectors" (1973: 85).

A commuted death sentence to life imprisonment provides the catalyst for a different McCune to emerge, one who relates personally to other inmates, who traps and trains rats as pets, seeks correspondence with private citizens and ministers, and makes character studies of those around him. Within such a context he develops the perspective to relate his experience on paper, and ultimately accepts an association with a journalist, who makes his account accessible to us.

As limited as these three autobiographical accounts may be, they certainly expose as highly questionable the long-standing assumption, already challenged by Bogdan and Taylor (1976), that the mentally retarded are incapable of reflecting upon or constructing a coherent account of their lives.

THE LIFE HISTORY METHOD: ITS APPLICATION AND RELEVANCE TO RETARDATION RESEARCH

As a method in anthropology, the life history has been distinguished from ordinary biographies or autobiographies primarily because anthropologists worked most frequently with nonliterates — persons who, because they could not write, rendered their account through a second person (Kluckhohn, 1945; Langness, 1965; Langness and Frank, 1981). The most significant aspect of this is that life histories, unlike other biographical accounts, are by nature *collaborative* and are essentially the creation of two minds working together (Frank, 1979; Kennann, 1984). In the blending of "the consciousness of the investigator and the subject", it may not be possible to completely "disentangle" such personal threads (Frank, 1979; Langness and Frank, 1981). However, what life histories lack in "pure" introspection they make up for by providing an insider's view that simply cannot be otherwise obtained. The anthropological life history is therefore an ideal method for gaining an insider's perspective on living the life of a mentally retarded person, especially in view of the fact that the retarded are frequently nonliterate and that so few true autobiographies of the retarded are presently available.

Our work has begun to suggest the importance of the general and more specific perspectives afforded by the life history approach.[3] At the very least, life histories provide a broader description of those who have been labeled "mentally retarded" in our society. Through life histories we are able to view single individuals through time in their various roles as family members, students, clients of the delivery system, employees, spouses, and even parents, and can create composite portraits of them that are far more complete than the profiles suggested by test scores, questionnaires, and ordinary interviews. In addition to holistic description, however, life histories offer us their unique "insider's perspective" on mental retardation by granting the retarded individuals a voice and allowing them to share their own perception of their roles and experiences. As Bogdan (1977) has already stressed, this emic view of retarded individuals is invaluable to both a qualitative appreciation of mental retardation and a more complete understanding of the social institutions of which retarded individuals are a part.

While such ends are sufficient in themselves to justify the use of the life history method, the collaborative nature of this technique allows for further and deeper understandings. Though the life history method begins with autobiographical accounting, the researcher, too, plays an active role by encouraging the informant to provide a commentary on events as they are brought to light and, further, by analyzing this commentary to obtain understandings that may not be a part of the individual's emic view. One aspect of our work with Ted Barrett (Whittemore, this volume), a mildly retarded man with whom extensive life history work has been done over a more than 15 year period (Edgerton, 1967), provides a model of this process. When we asked Mr. Barrett to shoot Super-8 movies of his world, independently, and to therefore visually expound on his daily life, we ended up scanning through his eyes the inner city environment in which he lives. On the film there is buffoonery, visual recognition of a cohort of significant others, and extensive urban landscapes containing a myriad of human and material details. In and of itself the film portrays a quality of life and an expressedly emic viewpoint that is vital to our understanding of how such individuals exist. But in our presence, while viewing his own cinematographic efforts, Barrett moved beyond the merely descriptive dimension by providing comments on his efforts. In these comments on the visuals, he gave renewed attention to the differences and the detail which he had tried to capture on film, criticized himself for his lack of technical clarity, and expressed disturbed concern over objects in his portrayed environment which of themselves or in context did not entirely make sense to him. As researchers, we attended carefully to his commentary, seeking the highly personal feelings about competence and well-being in the community that were embedded in his discussion of the "slice of life" he had captured. It was in the nexus of the "visual" and "commentary" that his own ruthless self-doubt and criticism emerged. Thus, his commentary furthered our understanding of his view of the world, his personality, and how both serve as adaptive mechanisms which he employs as he negotiates an exceedingly complex and difficult environment. In the course of a "critical review" of the interface between life events and their personal interpretation, the researcher comes to understand the individual in a way that the individual him or herself probably cannot.

We see, then, that in addition to general description, a life history effort lends itself to a uniquely detailed description built both upon the emic view of the individual and the analytic and reportorial skill of the researcher. It is from this broad descriptive base that our own life history work has moved on to demonstrate an additional series of more specific analytic benefits attached to the use of this method. These benefits are enumerated in the remainder of this paper and in the papers which follow.

Within anthropology, the life history method was one answer to a paradox built into the nature of the field work endeavor and its final product. Through prolonged and intensive contact with the individuals of a group, anthropologists seek an understanding of the group's culture and social institutions. Resulting monographs ordinarily deal predominantly with the life of the group as a whole with far less attention given to the manner in which modal social forms shape and are shaped by the very individuals who provide an understanding of them. In response to a growing frustration over the "disappearing individual", the life history has emerged as a dynamic means through which the articulation and interaction of the individual with his or her larger social context can be explored.

In much the same manner, life histories of mentally retarded individuals can serve to reconcile a wide range of individual and social frames of analysis mediating between the individual and his or her social context. For instance, a number of explanations have been offered in the attempt to come to grips with the "cause and nature" of mental retardation. One body of literature asserts that mentally retarded people are disabled because of pathological genetic structures (Goddard, 1912; Jensen, 1970; Reed and Reed, 1965) or because of anoxia-related brain damage (Richmond, Tarjan and Mendelsohn, 1965). Another suggests that etiology lies at the level of familial/social deprivation (Farber, 1968; Hurley, 1969). Yet another finds the key in the process by which individuals are labeled by social institutions and then pressured to act in ways consistent with the behavior imputed by that label (Braginsky and Braginsky, 1971). Typically, each body of literature cites other viewpoints but proclaims the overriding significance of its own perspective, thereby limiting itself to one primary aspect of a rather complex reality. The life history method, being the best if not only means by which an individual can be examined holistically, and through which the operation of diverse variables can be examined concurrently, stands as an avenue to resolving this analytic confusion. A good life history manages to isolate an individual's unique perspective on his or her biology and personality, and to tease out the reciprocal relations between these aspects (which define him or her as an individual) and each of those social and cultural contexts in which the individual interacts — family, work, community, and society. Here is the foundation for an eclectic model of disability and an alternative to the fragmented and incomplete models that tend to arise from analysis limited to only one plane to human experience.

Betsy Valen's life history (Koegel, 1981) for example, although only summarized here, suggests the manner in which all of these frames of analysis interact and how life history helps set the stage for a more dynamic understanding of mental retardation. From a very early age, Betsy was observed to be slightly slower than most children and certainly slower than her three older and four younger siblings. Whether this "slowness" resulted from very high fevers that accompanied a severe bout with pneumonia at age 16 months, from some undetected birth related trauma, from genetic endowment, or merely from position on the lower end of a normal intelligence distribution is unclear. What *is* clear is that Betsy's slowness exists as a biological fact which exerted a profound influence on the shape of her life despite the fact that her family did not apply the "mental retardation" label to her. An older sister recalls that as a "slower" member of a large and active family, Betsy receded quietly into the background, withdrawing from competition within her family and making no demands. Betsy's adaptive strategy, in turn, was apparently reinforced when family members found it easier to deal with a passive, quiet Betsy who asked for no attention or aid rather than to respond to a demanding Betsy who insisted on support when attempting to hold her own. From the natural fact of Betsy's "slowness" arose a unique interactive social process, the consequences of which encouraged a certain passivity in Betsy, restricted the level of her exposure to socio-emotional contact, and deprived her of experience in the practical tasks of daily existence. However, though as a youth she had been placed in a special school, Betsy had not yet attracted a label of being mentally retarded. Her entry into the official ranks of the mentally retarded did not take place until her mid-twenties. Following a nervous breakdown, Betsy had been employed in a workshop for individuals with a variety of handicaps. Then, a move from one board and care facility to another precipitated her relocation to a workshop servicing the mentally retarded exclusively. As far as anyone can tell, the workshop transfer was one of convenience; the shop was chosen for its proximity to Betsy's residential facility despite the fact that she had not been labeled mentally retarded. When Betsy's funding through the Department of Rehabilitation (a funding source for all disabled individuals) was terminated however, her case, along with others, was routinely sent over to the Regional Center for the Developmentally Disabled. Because Regional Center routinely funded this workshop's clients and because a psychiatrist from CCSS (Continuing Care Services Section, the agency responsible for out-of-home placement of mentally ill and retarded individuals) subjectively evaluated Betsy as being mildly retarded, Betsy became a client of an agency solely responsible for the mentally retarded. All indications are that Betsy was labeled to expedite funding procedures and to justify her placement in the workshop reserved for the retarded. Years later, in fact, upon applying for funding for a rather expensive training facility, Betsy was retested, at which time she was no longer classified as retarded. The dramatic upheaval in Betsy's life which this administrative change precipitated was sufficient to elicit a complete psychotic break from which she has only recently recovered. The paper by Edgerton in this volume describes a similer case although the consequences were not quite so extreme.

While space does not allow Betsy Valen's life history to be presented in all its fascinating complexity, this portion of it does suggest how various levels of analysis are inextricably tied together. We see how the dynamic interaction between Betsy's biological "slowness", the demands of her family/community, and the adaptive strategies (e.g., personality and demeanor) she developed to cope with those demands feed into a mutually reinforcing, spiralling process that serves to inhibit Betsy's socio-emotional growth and her experience in the practicalities of social existence. We see how these sociobiological determinants leave Betsy an unlikely candidate for the service delivery system which then contributes as well to the ongoing process, reinforcing her patterns of passivity and dependency, structuring her life experiences, and profoundly shaping her competence. How can one explain the nature of Betsy's unique position in her family without considering her biological background? How can one explain her entrance into the system in the first place without paying heed to her unique socialization experience? How can one understand the full nature of what is called her "limited intelligence" without considering the way her family and the delivery system have limited her experience? The answers to all of these questions are inextricably tied together; it is within the kind of holistic approach which life history analysis offers that answers to all can be most satisfactorily obtained.

In portraying the life of Doug Valpey, another individual in our pool of life history candidates, Turner (1980) found a similarly complicated portrait of disability. A multitude of historical facts, including familial transience and size, spotty educational opportunity, economic deprivation, and uninspired social workers could be recalled by Doug and appear to have contributed to what he had come to accept as his disability. After a lengthy collaboration and friendship between Valpey and Turner, the former agreed to a psychological retest of his abilities. As is the case surprisingly often, this testing reclassified Doug as not retarded by delivery system standards. Quite interestingly, Doug's "commentary" changed radically on the basis of this new and startling evidence. Whereas during the time that he had accepted the mental retardation label, he had retrospectively interpreted many of his competencies as an effort to prove to people that the retarded, himself included, were capable of more than what they were given credit for, he subsequently reinterpreted these actions as an attempt to prove to other people that indeed he was not and never had been retarded. As with Ted Barrett, the reflexive aspect of the life history enterprise is shown to offer a wealth higher level understandings. Thus, Valpey and Turner's collaboration provides a remarkable opportunity for viewing disability and competence as dialectical phenomenon, open to the influence of many variables. The life history method, open to a variety of analytic frames, can suggest that the "truth" of disability lies in the *interaction* of influences to which the individual as both biological and social organism is exposed over the course of his or her life.

The cases of Betsy and Doug suggest yet another advantage of the life history method. Synchronic research has already revealed how an individual may be considered retarded in one setting (e.g., the classroom) but normal in another (e.g., the ethnic neighborhood) at the same point in time (Henshel,

1972; Mercer, 1973). Life histories, with their expressedly diachronic view, indicate in an equally clear manner that mental retardation is not always or necessarily a static, unchanging role assumed by an individual for life. Rather, it is a category in and out of which one can move over the course of time as a result of changing circumstances. Betsy and Doug are not alone in revealing the flexibility of mental retardation role assumption. Faith Castellana is one of many we have followed over time who has gone through similar status changes. Labeled retarded for all of the years she remembers, Faith attended special education classes, participated in leisure clubs for the mildly retarded, and was trained for hospital work in a program geared to the developmentally disabled. Marriage and childbirth, however, moved her further away from this world and closer to a self-image as a normal individual. In fact, she eventually had herself re-tested, and scored sufficiently high on an I.Q. test so as to allow her to discard the "retardation" label.

The processual, longitudinal nature of the life history method and the depth of the description it provides further highlights the limited value of the tools — test scores, questionnaires, sketchy case studies — typically used by those serving the retarded. Such tools by themselves simply do not and cannot predict competence and adaptational success (Cobb, 1972; McCarver and Craig, 1974). For example, a recent social worker evaluation characterizes Betsy Valen as "a rather withdrawn, complaining, anxious individual who has a great need for structure . . . who seeks to be dependent upon others; tends to withdraw from situations which are threatening or challenging and sees herself as quite inadequate in solving the problems of everyday living". Betsy does indeed manifest these qualities. What such a report cannot tell us, and what Betsy's life history *does* suggest, is that these presumed "deviant" behavioral characteristics (submissiveness, dependence, obsequiousness, fear of conflict) are adaptive strategies which Betsy has adopted in response to a peculiar set of life circumstances. Betsy's own account of her life and the perspectives offered by those who have played a significant role in their life consistently demonstrate the manner in which her passivity and dependence have been reinforced as coping strategies. Likewise, her history reveals in an equally consistent manner that conflict is seldom resolved. Compliance, dependence, and avoidance of threatening situations thus take on a new meaning when viewed within the diachronic context of her life.

Through Betsy's case an intensive look at one individual's life history reveals how behavior patterns that might be facilely explained in terms of individual handicap may sometimes prove to be of the utmost importance. Ted Barrett's history even more clearly indicates that behavior, which in service agency reports appears bizarre, may be understood as a successful adaptation to a tough, marginal life. Ted's Thematic Apperception Tests (as analyzed blindly by a clinical psychologist) portray him as isolated, with feelings of inadequacy and as having a history of arid family relationships. He is described as being immobilized in solving problems, responding to stress in relationships by backing off, and as favoring safe ground through indecisiveness. His hostility is seen to be repressed. He is described as not a verbal problem solver and as one who works with the authorities but characteristically exhibits a "macho" orientation in doing so. But what an extensive review of his life course reveals is that while such results accurately touch upon important themes in Ted's life, the test does not delineate the functional value of such traits to a man who has lead a remarkably healthy, independent life in the midst of the stressful and threatening inner city of Los Angeles for more than 20 years. In addition to failing to assess the operational value of certain characteristics in terms of long-term adaptive strategies for community life, projective tests, I.Q. tests, and even brief case histories cannot reveal the mosaic pattern of competence and individual strengths that counter-balance the more evident deficiencies of those who are called "retarded".

More specifically, in terms of adaptation, the life history's focus on socialization over the life course can reveal how certain forms of "retarded" behavior may better be understood as functions of social learning, denied opportunity (i.e., lack of practice in conventional roles and settings), or adjusted expectations emerging from assumptions of pervasive incompetence. That incompetence can be *created* as a result of such factors is clearly illustrated by what may appear to be a relatively innocuous incident in John Hamlin's past (Koegel, this volume). Currently 26, John vividly recalls an evening five years earlier when his parents and brothers returned home from dining out only to find him sitting in his "dad's chair" with his feet propped up on the coffee table and for the first time, with a drink in his hand. While seemingly unconcerned, John's father proceeded to join him, offering him unlimited quantities of a variety of alcoholic beverages in a calculated effort to make John dreadfully ill. He was more than successful in his mission. John was confined to his bed for the next two days, having only enough energy to occasionally fill the pail his mother had strategically place by his side. Referring to the event as a "cure", John's father points to its efficacy (John turns his nose up at the offer of a drink) and maintains that he applied the same cure to John's older brother. Actually, the approach to John's brother had been radically different. The latter, a fledgling musician, had, at age 16, begun playing parties at which alcohol was readily available. Concerned that he would drink more than he should to be able to drive safely, John's father had his nonretarded son carefully monitor his feelings as they drank together so that he could establish a safe "limit" and be fully aware of what he could handle. In other words, John's brother was given the opportunity to learn to handle drinking maturely and responsibly. Subtly communicated to him was the fact that he was an adult and deserved to be treated as such. John, on the other hand, was conditioned out of a desire to drink and was denied the opportunity to learn appropriate drinking behavior. Subtly communicated to him was the fact that he was not an adult, did not deserve to be treated as one, and should not think of himself as one. The consequences of this lesson thus go far beyond John's aversion to drinking, though this is itself stigmatizing in the social circles in which his family travels. Of crucial importance here is the fact that John and his brother have been raised according to a separate and markedly different set of "rules". While John's early behavioral and academic problems might have justified a special set of rules at certain times and in certain domains, this critical event suggests a generalizing effect: differential application of rules has taken place in areas that need not be affected by John's presumed disabilities but that *are* ultimately affected as a result of the attitudes and assumptions organized around the perception of John as a "handicapped" individual. Other examples of this phenomenon exist both in the course of John's life and in the lives of others with whom we have worked. While some individuals may repress and thus fail to discuss such incidents, the life history method is more likely to obtain these kinds of data than less qualitative, longitudinal, and intensive methodologies.

One problem with a single emic perspective is that by definition such a view is highly individual, personal, and may explain but one life. At first glimpse then, its rewards may seem pale in light of the amount of time involved in the generation of a life history and in the intensity demanded from both the retarded individual and a collaborator during its formulative course. And yet, as we have noted above, despite the unfortunate absence of the view of the retarded themselves in the family and social service based biographical literature, the virtue of the collected body of such works lies in the recurring patterns of grief, struggle, and occasional symbiosis which do emerge from these accounts. While the risk is that a single life history may be too specific, a collection of such accounts may establish themes and/or patterns of vital importance to professional and community understanding and response to mental disability.

An example of such an emergent theme is the fact that what is taken to be a usual "arc of life" (Cain, 1964) for most "normal" individuals just does not describe what we see in the life histories of the retarded. Adult years for the retarded are characterized by marginal, transient membership in the occupational, familial, and community traditions of social interaction which in adulthood are "normally" the firm foundations for individual initiative and freedom. In the retarded individual's life course, age is not typically pivotal in perceived abilities and individually accepted privileges. The assumption is, of course, that the retarded simply remain children throughout their life span. What then *are* the developmental cornerstones which do give direction to such lives? Is there a developmental cycle to mild retardation which, in the form of personal "passages" or critical incidents, shapes the needs, motives and intentions of the retarded individual? In comparing such patterns with "normal" developmental expectations, what is there that prevents normal attainment of social development? Such things as familial transience, presumed accidental trauma, institutionalization, and contact with a social service delivery system are common experiences of significance to the mildly retarded. What we expect is that attention to these life events will diminish the distracting and ubiquitous issue of natal or childhood etiology, something which tends to be the product of the clinical "case history" approach to disability, and inspire full understanding of the consequences and causes and nature of disability within a life in process. Korbin's paper in this volume speaks to the discontinuity in development that increasingly feeds on itself as the retarded person matures.

This is not to argue that by posing singular exceptions to a homogeneous conceptual category of "retardedness", individual portraits have not served their purpose. It is individual life courses which, in our experience with this population, highlight the heterogeneity of individual appearance, residental history, past employment or prospects for work, emotional response to personal limitation or adversity, and highly variant sexual experience. Such "exceptions to the rule" render categorical approaches to retardation inadequate. Thus, for all the similarity of past events that may be found in the lives of the retarded, the life history focus can inform us of the highly variable manner in which the retarded have responded to these crucial life events. Certainly it is knowledge of such responsiveness within the life course which is central to research and community concern over adaptive success for the mildly retarded.

All of the points which we have enumerated above on the descriptive and evaluatory significance of the life history approach have been oriented toward the concerns of the scientific and social service communities. But they have not necessarily been pertinent to the members of the community itself. We feel, as does Bogdan (1977), that the accessibility of the disabled experience to the community at large will also be best served by an insider's view. Certainly the popularity of recent television specials on the lives and trials of the handicapped, and the media attention given Robert Meyers' *Like Normal People* (1978) and Barry Morrow's fine motion picture, *Bill*, (for which Mickey Rooney won an Emmy, indicate lay interest in the sensitizing experience of such personal accounts. We hope that the papers in this collection will do likewise.

Perhaps more importantly, we must not ignore the impact which the construction and dissemination of a retarded individual's life history may have on him or herself. After all of our scientific justification for the proliferation of these histories, we feel there is a compelling argument for the life story affording some retarded individuals a monumental opportunity to entertain, engage in, and identify with the process of making their own worthwhile contribution to a literature of direct bearing on their future. Indeed, despite ethical argument for the protection of subjects' privacy, we find it a compelling fact that Ted Barrett insists we no longer use his pseudonym and we honor his story by not disguising his name. We are made very aware of how committed Ted has become, and how urgently we feel about the task of making his, and our, unique contribution.

ACKNOWLEDGEMENT

A previous version of parts of this paper was published as Working Paper # 12, Socio-Behavioral Group, Mental Retardation Center, School of Medicine, University of California, Los Angeles. This research was made possible in part by NICHD Grant No. HDO 9474—02. It is part of a larger research project at UCLA, "The Community Context of Normalization", under the supervision of Robert B. Edgerton. We would like to thank Robert B. Edgerton and Gelya Frank for their comments during the preparation of this paper.

NOTES

1. Our search of the literature for biographical data on the mentally retarded has been comprehensive although there are a few relatively obscure references we have been unable to locate. We believe that the materials we have reviewed are representative of what is available even though not absolutely complete. (From 1916–1919, *The Psychological Clinic* [Lightner Witmer, ed.] published several brief case reports and clinical follow-up accounts which are not included in this review.)
2. The recent paper by Stanovich and Stanovich, "Bibliography of Writings by Mentally Handicapped Individuals", came to our attention during final draft preparation of this paper. We find some overlap with works we have mentioned and welcome the journal references of which we were not aware. Stanovich and Stanovich include Deacon (1974), which we had chosen to omit because of the concomitant physical handicap which larely colors this autobiographical effort, and yet do not include McCune (1973). Similarly, it seems that if Stanovich and Stanovich cite Braginsky and Braginsky (1971) *Hansels and Gretels* and Edgerton (1967) *The Cloak of Competence*, the failure to mention Henshel *The Forgotten Ones* (1972) and Mattinson's *Marriage and Mental Handicap* (1970) is a regrettable oversight.
3. The Community Context of Normalization Study has followed a cohort population of 48 individuals on a twice a month basis for the last three years. These individuals, ranging in age from 19 to 49 years, have all been labeled mentally retarded at some point in their lives but have been identified by professionals in the community service delivery system as possessing the potential for independent community living. Through the use of a naturalistic, qualitative methodology, i.e., one which attempts to observe and understand these adults in the context of their day-to-day lives, the study has sought to isolate factors which either help or hinder mildly retarded individuals to achieve normal lives within their communities. This research grew out of Robert B. Edgerton's pioneering study for *The Cloak of Competence* (1967).

REFERENCES

Begab, M. J. and Richardson, S. A. (eds.)
   1975 *The mentally retarded and society: A social science perspective.* Baltimore: University Park Press.
Bodgan, R.
   1977 *Voices: First person life histories as a method of studying retardation.* Unpublished manuscript presented at the 101st Annual Convention of the American Association on Mental Deficiency, New Orleans, June.

Bogdan, R. and Taylor, S.
    1976 The judged, not the judges: An insider's view of mental retardation. *American Psychologist, 31* (1): 47—52.
Braginsky, D. D. and Braginsky, B. M.
    1971 *Hansels and Gretels.* New York: Rinehart and Winston.
Buck, P. S.
    1950 *The child who never grew.* New York: John Day Company.
Cain, L. D., Jr.
    1964 Life course and social structure. *In* R. E. L. Faris (ed.), *Handbook of modern sociology* (pp. 272—309). New York: Rand McNally.
Cassel, R. H.
    1948 The man who might have been — I. Trent. *The Training School Bulletin, 45* (6): 105—108.
Cassel, R. H.
    1948 The man who might have been — II. Ted. *The Training School Bulletin*, 46: 114—118.
Cobb, H. V.
    1972 *The forecast of fulfillment.* New York: Teacher's College Press, Columbia University.
Deacon, J. J.
    1974 *Joey.* New York: Charles Scribner's Sons.
Edgerton, R. B.
    1967 *The cloak of competence: Stigma in the lives of the mentally retarded.* Berkeley: University of California Press.
Edgerton, R. B.
    1975 Issues relating to the quality of life among mentally retarded persons. In M. J. Begab and S. A. Richardson (eds.), *The mentally retarded and society: A social science perspective.* Baltimore: University Park Press.
Farber, B.
    1968 *Mental retardation: Its social context and social consequences.* Boston: Houghton Mifflin.
Frank, G.
    1979 Finding the common denominator: A phenomenological critique of life history method. *Ethos, 7* (1): 68—94.
Goddard, H. H.
    1912 *The Kallikak family.* New York: MacMillan. (Republished by MacMillan, 1931 and by Arno Press, 1973).
Greenfield, J.
    1965 *A child called Noah: A family journey.* New York: Holt, Rinehart and Winston.
Henshel, A. M.
    1972 *The forgotten ones: A sociological study of Anglo and Chicano retardates.* Austin, Texas: University of Texas Press.
Hunt, N.
    1967 *The world of Nigel Hunt. The diary of a mongoloid youth.* Beaconsfield: Darwan Finlayson, Ltd.
Hurley, R.
    1969 *Poverty and mental retardation.* New York: Vintage Books.
Jensen, A. R.
    1970 A theory of primary and secondary familial mental retardation. *International Review of Research in Mental Retardation, IV*: 33—105.
Kennann, Kristina
    1984 *Time in her life: A Down's woman's personal account.* Doctoral Dissertation, Anthropology Department, University of California at Los Angeles.

Kluckhohn, C.
   1945 The personal document in anthropological science. *In* Gottschalk, L., Kluckhohn, C., and Angell, R., *The use of personal documents in history, anthropology, and sociology* (pp. 79—173). New York: Social Science Research Council.
Koegel, P.
   1981 Life history: A vehicle towards the holistic understanding of deviance. *Journal of Community Psychology,* 9: 162—176.
Langness, L. L.
   1964 Biography: A common denominator. Presented to Section H (Anthropology), American Association for the Advancement of Science, Montreal, December 26—31.
Langness, L. L.
   1965 *The life history in anthropological science.* New York: Holt, Rinehart and Winston.
Langness, L. L. and Frank, G.
   1981 *Lives: An anthropological approach to biography.* Novato, California: Chandler and Sharp.
Malinowski, B.
   1922 *Argonauts of the Western Pacific.* New York: E. P. Dutton and Company.
Mattinson, J.
   1970 *Marriage and mental handicap.* Barton Manor, St. Philips, Bristol: Bristol Type Setting Company, Ltd. (Also published in Pittsburg: University of Pittsburg Press).
McCarver, R. and Craig, E.
   1974 Placement of the retarded in the community: Prognosis and outcome. *In* N. R. Ellis (ed.), *International review and research in mental retardation* (Vol. 7). New York: Academic Press.
McCune, B.
   1973 *The autobiography of Billy McCune.* San Francisco: Straight Arrow Books.
Mercer, J. R.
   1973 *Labelling the mentally retarded.* Berkeley and Los Angeles: University of California Press.
Meyers, R.
   1978 *Like normal people.* New York: McGraw Hill.
Morrow, Barry
   1981 *Bill.* CBS Television Network: Alan Landsburg Productions. Peabody Collection, University of Georgia, Athens, Georgia.
Murray, D. C.
   1956 *This is Stevie's story.* Elgin, Illinois: Brethren Publishing House.
Nash, A. M.
   1949 Mentally deficient; pseudo-socially successful: The boy who never grew up. *The Training School Bulletin, 46* (2): 20—28.
Reed, E. W. and Reed, S. C.
   1965 *Mental retardation: A family study.* Philadelphia: W. B. Saunders.
Richmond, J. B., Tarjan, G. and Mendelsohn, R. S.
   1965 *Mental retardation.* The American Medical Association.
Seagoe, M. V.
   1964 *Yesterday was Tuesday, all day and all night: The story of a unique education.* Boston: Little, Brown and Company.
Stanovich, K. E. and Stanovich, P. J.
   1979 Speaking for themselves: A bibliography of writing by mentally handicapped individuals. *Mental Retardation, 17* (2): 83—89.
Turner, J. L.
   1980 Yes I am human: Autobiography of a "retarded career". *Journal of Community Psychology, 8:* 3—8.

BIBLIOGRAPHY

Abraham, W.
   1958   *Barbara: a prologue.* New York: Rinehart and Company.
Anderson, C. M.
   1963   *Jan, my brain damaged daughter.* Portland: The Durham Press.
Deacon, J. and Roberts, E. I.
   1977   I will. *Special Children, 3* (2): 44—68.
Dixon, G.
   1945   Best world for Johnny. *Texas Outlook, 38*: 14.
Elliot, M. K.
   1950   Billy: A boy in the special class. *Understanding the Child, 19*: 123—126.
Elliott, M. K.
   1952   Virginia: A girl in the special class. *Understanding the Child, 21*: 116—117.
Frank, J. L.
   1975   Normalization — Marc, a young man I'll never forget. *Mental Retardation, 13* (3): 25.
Greenfield, J.
   1978   *A place for Noah.* New York: Holt, Rinehart and Winston.
Health, S. R., Jr.
   1941   Making up for lost time, a case study. *The Training School Bulletin, 38*: 1—5.
Hill, M.
   1950   Corky's 'E'. *National Parents and Teachers Magazine*, 50: 30—32.
Jewell, E. J.
   1928   Eddie finds happiness. *The Training School Bulletin*: 129—133.
Keener, M. R.
   1952   The man who might have been — III. Jimmy. *The Training School Bulletin* 49: 3—7.
King, J.
   1969   *Duncan.* Wellington, Australia: A. H. and A. W. Reed.
Lauber, E. G.
   1955   The vocational placement of a mentally retarded boy: A case history. *The Training School Bulletin, 52* (3): 43—49.
Lee, C.
   1961   *The tender tyrant: The story of a mentally retarded child.* Minneapolis: Augsburg Publishing House.
Motte, N. and Motte, P.
   1956   *The hand of the potter.* London: Cassell and Company.
Neal, E.
   1962   *One of those children: The spastic brain-damaged.* New York: Taplinger Publishing Co., Inc.
President's Committee on Mental Retardation.
   1974   *MR 74: A friend in Washington.* (The Eighth Annual Report of the President's Committee on Mental Retardation, pp. 6—8).
Roberts, N. and Roberts, B.
   1968   *David.* Richmond, Virginia: John Knox Press.
Rogers, D. E.
   1953   *Angel unaware.* Westwood, New Jersey: Fleming H. Revell Company.
Turnbull, A. P. and Turnbull, H. R. (eds.).
   1978   *Parents speak out: Views from the other side of the two-way mirror.* Columbus, Ohio: Charles E. Merrill Publishing Company.

SARAH: THE LIFE COURSE OF A DOWN'S SYNDROME CHILD

He explained to me that it was a *raw shok* test. He sad pepul see things in the ink. I said show me where. He dint show me he just kept saying think imaggen theres something on the card. I tolld him I imaggen a inkblot. He shaked his head so that wasnt rite eather. He said what does it remind you of pretend its something. I closd my eyes for a long time to pretend and then I said I pretend a bottel of ink spilld all over a wite card. And thats when the point on his pencel broke and then we got up and went out. I dont think I passd the *raw shok* test. (pp. 2—3)

The test [TAT] looked easy because I could see the pictures. She said this test and the other one the *raw shok* was for getting persinality. I laffd. I tolld her how can you get that thing from cards that somebody spilld ink on the fotos of pepul you dont even no. She lookd angrey and took the picturs away. I dont care. I gess I faled that test too. (pp. 4—5)

Daniel Keyes (1959)
Flowers for Algernon

Glimpses into the feelings and thoughts of retarded individuals are rare. Novelist Keyes vividly portrayed what life might be for a retarded man aware of his limitations while anthropologist Edgerton (1967) has provided unique insights on the coping mechanisms used by borderline retarded persons to give the illusion of normalcy, to wear their "cloak of competence". Nevertheless, the emic world of retardation has been largely ignored.

Life histories have been proposed as a powerful means for understanding the emic perspective of culturally diverse peoples, important individuals, deviants, and the retarded (Kluckhohn, 1945; Langness, 1965; Langness and Frank, 1981; Whittemore, Koegel and Langness, 1980). While there are few life histories of retarded adults (Hunt, 1967; Langness and Frank, 1981; Segoe, 1964; Turner, 1978; Whittemore, Koegel and Langness, 1980), life histories of retarded children, and children in general, are virtually non-existent. A "life history" by its terminology implies that one has a life to recount. Life histories of children presumably have not been regarded as compelling in the same way as those of adults since in childhood one is at the start of their life story while by adulthood a more complete version can be told. However, children's views of their lives, if they could be obtained, would provide us with a valuable perspective. Policy decisions are made on the basis of a belief that some retarded individuals will be able to live relatively independently as adults, yet little is known of the course of events that enhance or impede such development. Prospective life course data should hold considerable promise for identifying the factors that contribute to successful versus unsuccessful adaptations among the retarded.

This chapter will explore what can be learned about the adaption and adjustment of a handicapped child through the medium of a prospective life

19

L. L. Langness and H. G. Levine (eds.), Culture and Retardation, 19—32.

study of a child with Down's Syndrome. This child, Sarah (a pseudonym), was among the subjects of a larger research project aimed at assessing retarded children's competences in their home environments and how this corresponded with the profile obtained from school records and more formal testing procedures. Although Sarah's I.Q. was tested at 37 when she was nine years old, her activities outside of the testing situation belied such a low score. Since Sarah's articulation was largely incomprehensible, the material presented is not a life history in the strict sense of the term. Instead, data was gathered through participant observation in her home environment (Edgerton and Langness, 1978) and interviews with her parents and teachers. A telephone interview with and letter from Sarah's mother five years after the research project provided a longitudinal perspective on the life course development of this child.

RETARDATION AS AGE-COMPETENCE INCOGRUITY

A major criterion of mental retardation in our society is the discrepancy between chronological age and exhibited competence (R. B. Edgerton, personal communication, 1982) whether measured in terms of I.Q. scores or adaptive behavior scales (Meyers *et al.*, 1979). As an individual matures, he/she is expected to follow a trajectory of increasing skills and competence. While this development may be uneven, it nevertheless proceeds in the expected direction. In the case of the retarded, the trajectory is disrupted by a widening gap between chronological age and competence.

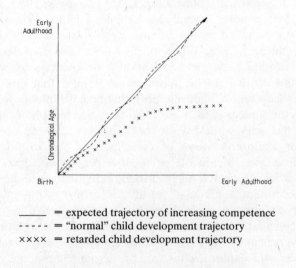

```
_____  = expected trajectory of increasing competence
- - - -  = "normal" child development trajectory
××××     = retarded child development trajectory
```

Fig. 1: Age-Competence Incongruence.

As an intellectually normal child begins to exhibit even the most rudimentary skills, others, particularly parents and teachers, rightfully expect that these skills are the precursors of subsequent development. There is little reason not to believe, barring accident or misfortune, that the trajectory of increasing competence will continue.

With retarded children, however, these expectations are thrown into disarray. Down's Syndrome infants display a normal course of motor development for approximately the first six months of life, after which development increasingly falls below the norm (Fisler, 1975; Share, 1975). As skills are accrued, even at a later age than the normal range, parents may interpret such development as a promising sign. This hopefulness is not necessarily unrealistic, but may be reflective of beliefs about the usual course of maturation. Glimmers of competence may lead parents to hope that the trajectory of development, while perhaps limited or delayed, will continue.

As retarded children's skills and competence grow increasingly out of synchronization with chronological age, problems are created both for parents (and other socialization agents) and for the retarded individual. Parents must reevaluate and restructure their perceptions of and hopes for the child. The retarded child, who at 6 or 8 was given great praise for riding a bicycle or counting to ten, may at 18 years of age still be riding a bicycle and counting to ten as his or her highest level of achievement. Behaviors that were viewed as precursors of skills in a younger child must come to be viewed as the plateau or end point in an older individual. Expectations are then sharply brought into focus with the reality of retardation.

SARAH

Sarah's parents were in their mid-40s when Sarah was born. They adopted a son approximately two years previously, assuming that after fifteen years of marriage they would not conceive. Sarah's parents were middle-class, practicing Catholics, with high school educations.

When Sarah was born, the physician told Mrs. J. that she had given birth to a "mongoloid idiot" who would probably live into her 20s but "never be able to do anything". The doctor's partner, however, said that Sarah would progress, but at a much slower rate than non-impaired children. Whenever possible, Mrs. J. took Sarah to the partner.

Sarah's parents were aware of the limitations of individuals with Down's Syndrome and that Sarah never would be able to live independently. Since they were older, they could not realistically assume that they would be able to care for her throughout her lifetime. They hoped that her brother would be able to support his future family and Sarah in a duplex-type living arrangement, or that Sarah would live and work in a sheltered environment. Sarah's parents were active in organizations for parents of retarded children, particularly Down's Syndrome children, and participated in school activities and in promoting religious education for retarded children. They considered themselves fortunate that Sarah was relatively bright and her behavior easy to manage in comparison to the other retarded children with whom they came into contact.

SARAH AT NINE YEARS OF AGE

At nine years of age, when first contacted, Sarah was an engaging child and one who seemed bound to be a "success story" for her parents and teachers. Sarah's parents felt that she would need supervision as an adult, but that she would be able to perform a routine job and use public transportation to and from work. While they acknowledged her handicap, they also felt that she could make a contribution, however small, as a productive member of society. Her parents felt that having a job was essential to any person's life, including the retarded. Sarah's teachers believed that she was a "good candidate" for sheltered independent living as an adult, and selected her to be among the first children "mainstreamed" from her TMR (trainable mentally retarded) school into a "regular" school.

Sarah displayed a range of competencies in her environment. She took long walks in the neighborhood with her dog, swam, rode her bicycle with training wheels, and sang along to records that she played on her record player. She went to the neighborhood store by herself and purchased snacks. She helped her mother perform tasks such as dusting and setting and clearing the table. She usually kept her toys and possessions in order, cleaning up her room after she was through playing.

Sarah could perform independently most self-care and hygiene tasks including bathing, hair combing and brushing of teeth. She could dress herself, being careful to put labels in the back. Sarah could recognize a few words and took weekly trips with her mother to the public library to check out books. She sat in her room "reading" these library books for hours. She could recognize letters and spell a few words, print the alphabet and her name, count to 20 (with some help), name colors, and recite her address and phone number. She would also recite lists of all the individuals living in her house, including the pets. At school, children were grouped according to their abilities and Sarah was in all of the highest groups; in language, math, physical education, and visual perception.

Mrs. J. reported that Sarah had always been "independent", wanting "to do things for herself". Mrs. J. and Sarah, for example, read together at bedtime. Sarah often insisted on reading aloud to her mother, turning the pages, pointing out pictures and words, and talking in her "garbled way" (according to Mrs. J.). This made the bedtime routine much longer than when Sarah's mother read. While this may be the case for many young children, Sarah's mother had less reason to expect that it would change as her child matured.

It was not always an easy matter for Sarah's parents to encourage or allow independent behavior. While Sarah was competent at finding her way around her environment, she was not consistently aware of time constraints. As she left on her walks, she would say to her mother "dark" and Mrs. J. would respond, "no, before dark". The ability to consistently return home when it was about to turn dark was often beyond Sarah. On the few occasions that Sarah was not home by dark, Mrs. J. reported being worried and frantic. Each time Sarah was located, she was walking her dog and seemingly unconcerned about the darkness. Mrs. J. reported that these incidents made it hard for her to let Sarah go for walks alone but she felt it was important to allow her to function as independently as possible.

Sarah's behavior on walks was not free from problems. Mrs. J. reported that Sarah ambled along slowly, looking at everything, such that strangers often assumed she was lost. Sarah had a bracelet with her name, address, and phone number, and Mrs. J. sometimes received calls saying that Sarah had been "found". An elderly man, upon "finding" Sarah, once angrily told Mrs. J. that "a child like that" should not be allowed out on her own. Mrs. J. pointed out, equally angrily, that Sarah had the right to enjoy the neighborhood like anyone else. Additionally, Sarah did not always obey the rules of privacy and property on her walks. Mrs. J. received complaints from the neighbors that Sarah stood at the windows of homes to watch what was transpiring inside. Mrs. J. repeatedly told Sarah not to do this, but often the smudges from window screens on Sarah's nose gave her behavior away. Sarah would also pick up pretty stones from people's rock gardens or pick their flowers to bring home to mother. Mrs. J. felt that this behavior, unlike the window-peeping, was easier for Sarah to control.

Mrs. J. also had fears about the dangers of Sarah being out alone since she was vulnerable to molestation. She felt that the dog would be a slight deterrent, but that, as a parent of a retarded child, she was at the mercy of strangers. Her child would be unable to protect herself, if indeed she realized what was happening to her.

While stereotypes of Down's Syndrome children as happy, affectionate, and easy-going are overdrawn (Edgerton, 1975; Silverstein, 1964), Sarah was basically an even-tempered and pleasant child. She displayed a range of moods, and was not consistently happy or affectionate. Her family was not physically demonstrative and neither was she. Sarah expressed anger and fought as did her intellectually normal older brother. On one occasion he teased her and turned off her favorite television program. She seemed to take it in stride and went into her room, only to reappear later and hit him when he wasn't looking. She could sometimes wait patiently. At other times, such as when Polaroid pictures were being taken, she would stamp her foot and holler her objections at having to wait for the picture to develop.

Sarah displayed an ability to engage others socially. A consistent report from her school was that she got along well with peers and teachers. She also got along well with other children in the neighborhood. Sarah participated in the Special Olympics, displaying behavior that has become a cliché in media portrayals or retarded children. She was close to the lead in her race when she spotted her parents and brother in the stands. She stopped to smile, wave, and call to them before proceeding to finish almost in last place.

Sarah also exhibited empathy in response to other's pain. When her friend scraped her foot on the concrete in their backyard, Sarah immediately called for her mother to get a band-aid and examined the scrape, made sympathetic "ouching" sounds, and put an arm around her friend. At school, Sarah's teachers reported that when one of her classmates was punished and made to sit on the bench during recess, Sarah was always the first student to go to the culprit and put an arm around his/her shoulders.

Sarah's poor articulation seemed to be her major problem. The literature more often is cognizant of problems that parents, teachers, siblings, and peers have in understanding the retarded than of problems that the retarded have in making themselves understood. Sarah's family had mixed success in understanding her speech. They would sometimes be able to interpret long stories she told about past events and at other times unable to understand what she was saying. Their interpretation of stories was undoubtedly based to some extent on shared context such that interpretation of specific words was made easier. Her teachers also were able to understand her only sporadically, but with increasing success after they had time to accommodate to her in their classrooms. Interestingly, Sarah had a playmate who also had a speech impairment but these two children almost always seemed able to verbally communicate. They regularly conversed on the telephone, coordinating plans about activities and where to meet. Sarah regularly followed her phone calls with Jennifer by accurately telling her mother either that Jennifer was coming over or that she was going to her house. Sarah and Jennifer also coordinated plans about play materials. Jennifer would often arrive with the same or coordinating objects, for example play dough to go with the cookie cutters that Sarah had readied. The two children immediately would set to work. Price-Williams and Sabsay have discussed the communicative abilities of Down's persons in an institutionalized environment (1979). Kennann has discussed at length how she became able to communicate more effectively with such a person (1984).

Sarah had demonstrable communication. Sometimes utterances of several words would be responded to while at other times a single word was unintelligible. Her frustrations were often evident on the occasions when, after several repetitions of the same phrase, she would scream something unintelligible, but different, and storm away from her listener. On one occasion, Sarah told me on the telephone, "I have on gaucho pants". Not quite believing that I heard correctly, I repeated her statement with a question mark on the end. Sarah confirmed by saying yes. To check, I then asked her what color they were and she responded that they were brown. Sarah then uttered another long phrase that I was unable to understand after four repetitions. She then slammed the telephone down on the table. When her mother picked up the telephone, she confirmed that Sarah was wearing the outfit reported. However, Mrs. J. also was unable to understand the second part of Sarah's conversation.

Sarah could also devise adaptations that allowed her to communicate when her speech was not understood. When her repeated statement that her brother was eleven years old was not understood, in exasperation she held up her two index fingers very close together, making a visual "11". This is consistent with other research that "brighter" Down's Syndrome children develop means of communicating with gestures (Share, 1975).

Differences between performance and competence take on particular importance among children such as Sarah. Although she was capable of counting, spelling her name, and reciting her address, she would sometimes balk at performing. This refusal to be "put through the paces" is familiar to all parents who attempt to proudly display their offspring's latest achievements. With retarded children, however, there is more difficulty in sorting our whether the child is actually unable to perform the requested tasks, or whether he/she simply does not want to comply. On one occasion, I brought a tape recorder to Sarah's house. Sarah was intrigued with the machine, wanting to play with it and operate it herself. In spite of her fascination with the tape recorder, I tried to get her to perform some skills so that I could record them. The following exchange ensued:

JK: Can you count to ten for me?
Sarah: Okay. One, two, three, four (pause).
JK: That's four, what comes next?
Sarah: Quiet! (to brother who was whispering, "what comes next?")
JK: Okay. Five.
Sarah: Five.
JK: Then what?
Sarah: Nine.
JK: Nine?
Sarah: Yeah. Nine.
Jk: Start over. Start over at one.
Sarah: One, two, three, four, five, six (pause).
JK: That's good. What comes after six?
Sarah: Nine.
JK: Seven.
Sarah: Seven.
JK: Then what?
Sarah: Nine.
JK: What about eight.
Sarah: Eight. .
JK: Then what?

Sarah: Nine.
JK: Then what comes after nine?
Sarah: (no answer)
JK: How old are you going to be on your birthday?
Sarah: (held up ten fingers)
JK: Yes, but what's that?
Sarah: Ten.
JK: Ten, that's right.
Sarah: (pointing to switch on tape recorder) What's that?
JK: That's the switch to make it start and stop.
Sarah: (pointing to "stop" on the tape recorder) Stop, s-t-o-p (spelling out
         the word).
JK: Good. Can you spell your name too?
Sarah: Sarah.
JK: Yes, Sarah, but how do you spell Sarah?
Sarah: (audible sigh) Nine. Come on (reaching for tape recorder).

Since I had observed Sarah count to ten and spell her name numerous times, her continuing response of "nine" made it easier to impute a motive of being exasperated with the task, or of just not feeling like performing. She was far more interested in playing with the tape recorder. While this is an indication of some level of awareness about manipulating people, it is not a measure of skills I was asking her to perform. A school psychologist who carried out Sarah's most recent psychological and cognitive testing wrote on her score sheet: "Sarah is a girl who likes to please when she can. She gets tired and often refuses to work in a teasing sort of way." Similarly, in a "bingo" game with pictures at Sarah's school, she repeatedly held her hand over the correct picture, shaking her head in the negative to refuse a bingo chip. This was apparently to prolong the game since she was the last one finished even though she could have made several "bingoes".

None of Sarah's skills and behaviors were particularly remarkable for a nine year-old child. They do seem to be, however, out of line with what would be expected on the basis of her I.Q. score of 37. This discrepancy, in combination with her engaging personality, made her prognosis seem bright.

SARAH AT FOURTEEN YEARS OF AGE

A telephone interview and a letter from Sarah's mother five years later, when Sarah was 14, provided a helpful longitudinal perspective. Many of Sarah's skills and activities had changed very little, and the prognosis was not as optimistic as when she was nine.

When Sarah was eleven years old, her family moved to another part of the state due to a change in her father's employment. Her parents believe that Sarah's new school for trainable mentally retarded students, as well as the facilities for retarded adults, are not as good as those available to them in their original community. The family returns to their original home in the summers and plans to move back permanently when Sarah's father retires.

Sarah's language remains difficult to understand and she continues to receive speech therapy. This inability to communicate presents increasing problems for Sarah's adjustment.

In her out-of-school hours, Sarah engages in much the same activities as when she was nine. She takes long walks with her dog, swims, rides her bicycle, listens to her record player, and reads the books that she and her mother get from the public library. One of the few changes in Sarah's activities is that she rides her bicycle without training wheels. Mrs. J. reported that this had been a difficult transition. Sarah refused to let her father or brother remove the training wheels from her bicycle. They finally did so without her consent. She then walked the bicycle rather than riding it. She refused all attempts to teach her to ride until suddenly, for reasons that are not entirely clear, she simply began to ride it. Her brother believes that Sarah was persuaded to ride the bicycle by the chiding of an older neighborhood child of whom she had always been particularly fond.

Sarah continues to go to the store after school and on weekends to purchase snacks for herself. Mrs. J. assumes that Sarah is doing so satisfactorily because there have been no complaints and the family is well known to workers in the neighborhood stores. As was the case when Sarah was nine, Mrs. J. asks her what she wants to buy and then gives her the correct amount of money. At nine, Sarah could discriminate between pennies and dimes, but confused nickels and quarters. This remains the case at 14. Because of her speech difficulties, the shopping process runs more smoothly when Sarah can point out or pick up her selection. When she needs to verbally request an item, Mrs. J. writes her a note to give the salesperson.

Sarah's reading skills have not improved substantially. When she was nine years old she could recognize a few words. On her tenth birthday she was given a first grade workbook and could recognize most of the words. This was regarded as a positive sign for her future achievement level. At 14, however, she was reading only at a second grade level, another example of how she increasingly loses ground as she matures.

By the nature of participating in activities structured by her school, Sarah has acquired some new skills. She is enrolled in an electronics program in which she is learning to perform sorting tasks in preparation for possible employment opportunities. She is also involved in a woodshop class, where she makes platters, plaques, and napkin holders, and in an embroidery class where she makes pillows. These handicraft items are brought home to her family.

Sarah's social skills and environment have changed markedly. She now displays more difficult behaviors and has fewer other children with whom to play and interact. She refuses to speak or attend to one of her teachers, even though she seemed to like her in past semesters. Sarah has started talking and muttering to herself at home, seeming to withdraw into a world increasingly of her own. One of Sarah's teachers recently reported that Sarah is also engaging in this behavior at school. Mrs. J. believes that this is the result of having no friends with whom to talk. It is also reasonable to suspect that this behavior fits Sarah's continued experience of not being able to make herself understood. This interpretation is supported by Sarah's changed behavior in reading with her mother. She and Mrs. J. continue to go to the library to check out books. One of Sarah's teachers suggested that Sarah read these books aloud to help improve her articulation. However, despite Mrs. J.'s urgings, Sarah refuses and instead sits in her room alone "reading". When she was younger, she was eager to read to her mother and others. It is likely that she is simply less willing to engage in a frustrating task and perhaps is increasingly aware of her handicap.

Sarah's interaction with neighborhood children has undergone significant alterations. She had been friends with Jennifer for many years, and they played together on an almost-daily basis. Jennifer was three years younger than Sarah, and also had a speech impairment. While their conversation was often unintelligible to others, they made telephone arrangements to meet at one or the other's house and conversed during their play. When Sarah was 14, however, she and Jennifer were no longer playing together. In Mrs. J.'s letter she wrote, "The last two summers while we were in [their original community] were kind of sad for Sarah. I noticed Jennifer stopped coming over and soon Sarah quit going to her house." Since Jennifer had articulation and language problems of her own, her mother did not feel that Sarah was a good influence or suitable playmate any longer. When she was nine, Sarah also spent time playing with a neighborhood toddler. Mrs. J. reported that the little boy's mother seemed quite comfortable with Sarah coming over and keeping the child entertained. Sarah also seemed to enjoy his toys and playing with him. However, once past toddlerhood, the boy did not want to play with Sarah, complaining that she was too big, but still didn't know how to play many games. At 14 she still doesn't know how.

Sarah's passing menarche also marked a change in her mother's perceptions of her. Mrs. J. did not know how to explain menstruation to Sarah, except to tell her that it would happen each month. Sarah was apparently undisturbed and able to take care of her hygiene independently. This pleased Mrs. J. who compared Sarah with another child at Sarah's school who had to stay home when menstruating. Mrs. J. said that she would have to stop thinking of Sarah as a baby and start dressing her accordingly. The clothes she sewed for Sarah were not very different from what they had been for a long time, with puffed sleeves in pastel colors and childish prints of flowers, children, or animals. Mrs. J. now felt these might be "too babyish". Infantilization of the retarded in terms of dress, with the incongruity of an adult wearing children's clothing, is, of course, very common, marks their stigma, and makes interaction problematical.

Menstruation, of course, also brings up issues of sex, marriage, and procreation (Ell, 1977). Mrs. J. is a practicing Catholic who sees marriage, sexuality and procreation as inextricably linked and does not want Sarah to marry because she believes the children will have Down's Syndrome. When Sarah was nine, she had a "boyfriend" at school who gave her presents and kissed her. When I ask Mrs. J. if Sarah had a "boyfriend" at her new school, Mrs. J. said that Sarah didn't seem to be much interested in this now.

Sarah's parents continue to place a high value on her future employment. Mrs. J. wrote in her letter, "I do think a job of some sort is necessary for anyone so they feel they are contributing something besides breathing free air". Her parents do not want her to work in a public place, for example in food service, because they feel that the retarded person always gets the "short end of the stick". They also do not want her to work in a hotel or motel as a housekeeper because there is too much "hanky panky" going on and the retarded are too easily sexually exploited. As when Sarah was nine, they continue to believe that she is capable of working in a sheltered workshop, and that this is the best solution. Sarah was receiving some training in electronic assembly at school and seemed to like and be competent at this type of work.

CONCLUSION

Assessment of Sarah would be likely to differ if made only at one point in time, either when she was 9 or when she was 14. The crucial issue is not the specific skills that she exhibits at any given point in time, but the increasing incongruity between chronological age and expected competence. If a nine year-old's reading skills are at a first grade, or six year-old level, there is less discrepancy, and thus less potential disturbance, than a fourteen year-old who is reading at a second grade, or seven year-old level. These types of increasing disparities have far-reaching effects, beyond how well a retarded child performs in school or on tests of intelligence and adjustment. They deeply affect interpersonal relations and impact on the retarded individual's self-perception. As the age-competence discrepancy looms larger and larger, skills that Sarah displayed at nine years of age are less impressive, if not entirely inappropriate, at fourteen or twenty-two or thirty. This creates problems for those who interact with Sarah. It creates problems for Sarah who, previously reinforced and praised for skills, is now regarded in a very different perspective. Much more careful attention should be given to this process. When do skills plateau or begin to decline? What are the concomitant changes in the perceptions and behaviors of the handicapped? What changes in attitude are involved and how are these communicated? How do these changes interact and feed on each other? Might there be ways of avoiding this?

Detailed contextual information must be gathered in attempting to answer these questions. Such studies need to consider the handicapped person's view as well as that of investigators and significant others. Information gathered through life histories and participant-observation will aid in formulating testable hypotheses about the neglected processes of socialization and evaluation.

Down's Syndrome provides an example of a distinction familiar to medical anthropologists between the terms "disease", which involves an impairment of organs or organ systems, and "illness" which involves the individual's perception of a culturally disvalued state (Eisenberg, 1977). Although early intervention can have a significant impact on the development of Down's Syndrome individuals (Hanson, 1981), its chromosomal abnormalities cannot be "cured" but only prevented with amniocentesis and elective abortion of a fetus with the disorder (Kaback and Leisti, 1975; Stein, 1975). However, the "illness" component, the disvalued state of Down's Syndrome, can be altered. Younger Down's Syndrome children who display only a few years' discrepancy between chronological age and competence become less and less acceptable as they mature and the age-competence incongruity increases. Thus, while the disease entity of Down's Syndrome remains constant, the illness component is likely to get worse.

Sarah's poor expressive language abilities would make an exploration of her self-concept problematical. It is, however, an interesting question. Nigel Hunt, a Down's Syndrome individual who wrote his autobiography, repeatedly heard his parents and others referring to him as a "mongol". He asked his grandmother just what a "mongol" was, and she responded that it was a person who lived in Mongolia (Hunt, 1967). Similarly, when a 40 year-old woman with Down's Syndrome went to Disneyland with her mother, they were asked at the admission gate, "a child or an adult?" The Down's Syndrome woman immediately replied, "an adult of course, can't you see?" When Sarah was nine years old, her teachers were discussing her activities with me in her presence. Sarah covered her face with her lunch pail. Her teacher asked if she was embarrassed that we were talking about her, and Sarah nodded and took her lunch pail away from her face. It is difficult to know how Sarah's perceptions of others' responses to her and their changing reactions as she grows older impact upon her life and adjustment. While this may be a matter of conjecture until we develop improved means for tapping the self-concept of retarded individuals, it is nevertheless and important area for inquiry.

A prospective study of the life course development of retarded individuals, with specific attention to the increasing discrepancy between chronological age and competence, could provide us with a perspective on how the pieces of a retarded individual's life may stay fairly constant but the changing holes into which they must fit make life problematical. As cultural expectations increase with age, performance must keep pace. If it does not and the gap widens, the stigma becomes more apparent and successful adaptation more difficult. One wonders, in our tests and assessment of Sarah if she, like Keyes' character Charley would like to tell us: "I coudnt werk the puzzeles so good because it was all broke and the peices coudnt fit in the holes" (1959, p. 5).

ACKNOWLEDGEMENT

This research was carried out under the auspices of a grant of the Mental Retardation Research Center, Neuropsychiatric Institute, University of California at Los Angeles, "Program for the Development of the Mentally Retarded" (HD 00540). I would like to thank R. B. Edgerton and K. Nihira for their support and suggestions while the research was being conducted; and L. L. Langness and J. K. Eckert for their helpful comments during the preparation of the manuscript. I would especially like to thank Sarah (a pseudonym) and her family for their generosity in allowing me into their lives.

REFERENCES

Crane, J. and Angrosino, M.
    1974   *Field projects in anthropology.* Morristown, New Jersey: General Learning Press.
Edgerton, R. B.
    1967   *The cloak of competence. Stigma in the lives of the mentally retarded.* Berkeley: University of California Press.
Edgerton, R. B.
    1975   Community attitudes and Down's Syndrome. *In* R. Koch and F. de la Cruz (eds.), *Down's Syndrome [Mongolism]. Research, prevention, and management* (pp. 180—190). New York: Bruner/Mazel.
Edgerton, R. B. and Langness, L. L.
    1978   Observing mentally retarded persons in community settings. *In* G. Sackett (ed.), *Observing behavior. Theory and application in mental retardation* (pp. 335—348). Baltimore: University Park Press.
Eisenberg, L.
    1977   Disease and illness. Distinction between professional and popular ideas of sickness. *Culture, Medicine and Psychiatry, 1*(1): 9—23.
Ell, J.
    1975   Sexuality in the mentally retarded. *In* R. Koch and F. de la Cruz (eds.), *Down's Syndrome [Mongolism]. Research, prevention, and management* (pp. 208—213). New York: Bruner/Mazel.
Fisler, K.
    1975   Mental development in Mosaic Down's Syndrome as compared with Trisomy 21. *In* R. Koch and F. de la Cruz (eds.), *Down's Syndrome [Mongolism]. Research, prevention, and management* (pp. 87—98). New York: Bruner/Mazel.
Hanson, M. J.
    1981   Down's Syndrome children. Characteristics and intervention research. *In* M. Lewis and L. Rosenblum (eds.), *The uncommon child* (pp. 83—114). New York: Plenum.
Hunt, N.
    1967   *The world of Nigel Hunt. The diary of a mongoloid youth.* New York: Garett Publication.
Kaback, M. and Leisti, J.
    1975   Prenatal detection of Down's Syndrome: Technical and ethical considerations. *In* R. Koch and F. de la Cruz (eds.), *Down's Syndrome [Mongolism]. Research, prevention, and management* (pp. 47—66). New York: Bruner/Mazel.

Keyes, D.
  1959 *Flowers for Algernon.* New York: Bantam Books.
Kennann, Kristina
  1984 *Time in her life: A Down's woman's personal account.* Doctoral dissertation.
Kluckhohn, C.
  1945 The personal document in anthropological science. *In* L. Gottschalk, C. Kluckhohn
         and R. Angell (eds.), *The use of personal documents in history, anthropology, and
         sociology, 53*: 78—173. Social Science Research Council Bulletin.
Langness, L. L.
  1965 *The life history in anthropological science.* New York: Holt, Rinehart and Winston.
Langness, L. L. and Frank, G.
  1981 *Lives. An anthropological approach to biography.* Novato, California: Chandler and
         Sharp Publishers.
Meyers, C. E., Nihira, K. and Zetlin, A.
  1979 The measurement of adaptive behavior. *In* N. R. Ellis (ed.), *Handbook of mental de-
         ficiency* (rev. ed.). New York: Lawrence Erlbaum.
Price-Williams, D. R. and Sabsay, S.
  1979 Communicative competence among severely retarded persons. *Semiotica, 26* (1, 2).
Segoe, M.
  1964 *Yesterday was Tuesday, all day and all night. The story of a unique education.*
         Boston: Little Brown.
Share, J. B.
  1975 Developmental progress in Down's Syndrome. *In* R. Koch and F. de la Cruz (eds.),
         Down's Syndrome [Mongolism]. Research, prevention, and management (p. 78—86).
         New York: Bruner/Mazel.
Silverstein, A. B.
  1964 An empirical test of the mongoloid stereotype. *American Journal of Mental
         Deficiency, 68*: 493.
Stein, Z.
  1975 Family planning as a method of prevention. *In* R. Koch and F. de la Cruz (eds.),
         Down's Syndrome [Mongolism]. Research, prevention, and management (pp. 67—
         77). New York: Bruner/Mazel.
Turner, J.
  1978 *Yes I am human: Autobiography of a retarded career.* Paper presented at the 77th
         Annual Meetings of the American Anthropological Association, Los Angeles, CA.
Whittemore, R., Koegel, P. and Langness, L. L.
  1980 *The life history approach to mental retardation.* (Working Paper No. 12). (Available
         from the Sociobehavioral Research Group, Mental Retardation Research Center,
         University of California, Los Angeles.)

SANDRA Z. KAUFMAN

LIFE HISTORY IN PROGRESS: A RETARDED DAUGHTER EDUCATES HER MOTHER

I sat at my desk and slipped the tape into the tape recorder. Pressing the "forward" button, I listened. A few seconds went by, and I heard my daughter's voice.

I moved out of my mom and dad's house when I was around 19 or 21. I began living on my own and I really liked it a lot. Then I met a guy through high school. We were friends for a whole year in school. And then we began dating each other and having a good time and seeing each other a lot, and I went over to his house a lot, and then he asked me to go to grad night, and I couldn't go to grad night because my brother was going to a school in Massachusetts, and I either had a choice of either going to my brother's graduation or my own graduation. And I told Edgar — that's the guy I'm going with — that I was going to my brother's graduation. Then when I got home from my trip with my mother and father, I was still living at home. I called Edgar up because it was near my birthday, and I asked him, "Do you want to go to Disneyland for my birthday?" and he said, "Hey, yeah, sure," and so we went. And then we went and picked him up at his house, his mom's house, and then we got . . . after we were all done at the very last ride at Disneyland, we went . . . that's when I was turning 20 or 21 . . . I don't remember exactly . . . he gave me a ring, a really beautiful butterfly ring. And he asked, said to me, "I think I love you". And I was really, really happy, very happy . . .

I was still living at home, (but) I moved out like 2 or 3 months later. And then when I moved out, I moved into a place that belonged to my grandmother. And she lended it to me for a hundred and fifty, I think it was . . . I don't remember exactly . . . and it was downstairs from where I'm living now. And where I'm living now is a lot bigger place. I got a lot more room.

I was working down on the beach at a restaurant. I was a short order cook. And during that time I was still going with Edgar, and he had great problems. He had very difficult problems. Number one, he didn't have a job. Number two, he didn't have any money on him. Number three, he was living at his older brother's house with his brother's girl friend. And they were feeding him, having him have a place to live. He had a job once where his brother was working. Then he gave it up because it was too dangerous. And he was bringing home some money and some income, but still he . . . it wasn't very much. He was feeling all put down, up tight and all riled in, and I felt sorry for him. And so when I was living downstairs, I was . . . he came over to see me. I was, like, feeding him, giving him money if he needed it. I was doing everything I could possibly do . . .

Colette's voice stopped. Edgar could be heard in the background telling her she had it all "backwards". She considered and agreed he was probably right. Nevertheless, Colette's memories of how their relationship began had been set down on tape, and our mother-daughter collaboration to document her life history had begun.

I had been inspired to begin the project for two reasons. One was its uniqueness. No other parent had ever employed research methods to piece together the life history of her retarded child. Many had written biographical accounts, but the viewpoint was always that of the parent. By contrast, I

L. L. Langness and H. G. Levine (eds.), Culture and Retardation, 33—45.
© 1986 *by D. Reidel Publishing Company.*

wanted to understand my daughter's perspective. I wondered what events she would single out as important and how she would interpret them (Langness and Frank, 1981; Turner, 1980).

The other purpose was to repair our relationship. It had not always been poor. The friction began when she reached adulthood. As she grew up, her father and I had worried about what would become of her when that time arrived, and because no one could tell us, our imaginations had run wild. We pictured her sitting in the dreary day-room of a state hospital drooling over a half-completed pot-holder, or we saw her following us around the house and becoming a burden to her younger sister and brother when we died.

But in the early 1960s, attitudes toward the retarded began to change. Gradually, owing to President Kennedy's particular interest and the civil rights movement in general, the concept of normalization evolved: the handicapped were to be helped to lead as normal lives as possible. In this climate our beliefs changed. We began to think that with careful preparation Colette could eventually live in a semi-sheltered arrangement.

Colette, however, had other ideas. By the time she was 20, her father and I realized we were rapidly losing control of her. While we struggled to instill money management practices and the wisdom of birth control, she continued to disappear overnight with Edgar and to squander the wages from her part-time job.

One day she abruptly announced that she had found a tiny apartment, and she moved out. Stunned, we reacted with conflicting emotions. Although we were relieved to be finished with the stormy scenes that had exhausted us all, and we were proud of her determination, we were also worried and exasperated. Even after we moved her into an apartment owned by her grandmother so she could be nearer us, she continued to harbor unemployed Edgar who gave every indication of being lazy and parasitic. Her meagre earnings from her job at the fast-food restaurant were simply not enough to support both of them. In addition, the possibility of pregnancy made us frantic. We predicted that by her premature departure she had surely sabotaged whatever chances she had for continuing independence.

Problems did indeed occur with fatiguing regularity. During troubled times she turned to us and we bailed her out, accompanying our rescue operation with interrogations and scoldings. Gradually, however, we began to hear from her less and less. When I phoned, she was reserved and distant. Yet when we did get together, I always reverted to my role as inquisitor and judge, and she retreated further into lies and half-truths. We were locked into adversary positions.

Perhaps attempting her life history would bring us together again, I thought. I had a tremendous hurdle to leap, however. Such a collaboration requires neutrality on the part of the investigator, yet I would be coming into the research situation not only emotionally involved but also quite used to expressing my opinions forcefully. Keeping my reactions to myself would be very difficult. If I could do so, however, enough rapport might be engendered that she would feel free to talk about her early years, and in the process our deteriorating relationship might well be reversed. Encouraged by these possibilities, I decided to give the project a try.

After a family dinner celebrating her 24th birthday, I asked Colette if I could talk with her a moment alone. In presenting my proposal I avoided the term "retardation" because of the stigma (Edgerton, 1967). Instead, I explained that the professors I work with[1] were interested in the stories of handicapped young people. I thought her story would be particularly interesting, and I wondered if she would let me write it. Any final copy would be read to her, I promised, and she could demand revisions or deletions.

Colette was barely able to pay attention to me, for the topic was of far less interest to her than my suddenly neutral demeanor. It unleashed a torrent of long-festering grievances over my insistence she not become pregnant. For 40 minutes I exhibited reassurance and sympathy while gently trying to ease the conversation back to my research. Colette said she would have to think about it.

A few days later she called to announce that she had decided to try it, but she wanted to talk into a tape recorder without my being present. I agreed, brought her the machine and a tape, and the result was her description of becoming involved with Edgar and of leaving home. Subsequent efforts on my part to elicit memories failed, however; she was uninterested and impatient with my asking questions concerning past events about which she insisted I was more knowledgeable than she.[2] Not only that, she proved so reactive to both the tape recorder and my pad and pen that I had to abandon them. In response, I changed my research goal and my method of recording. I would document two years of on-going history as she was experiencing them. Recall of earlier events would be captured as they spontaneously emerged, but they were no longer to be the focus. She and I would do whatever it is that mothers and daughters do together, except that I would listen and observe. My goal would be that of the ethnographer: to try to see the world as Colette sees it. Field notes would be recorded either surreptitiously or immediately after our interactions.

The study has now been completed, and I am beginning to organize my field notes documenting over 600 phone calls and in-person contacts made during the two years and four months of our project. As I re-read them, I have become aware that my relationship with Colette has undergone a transformation. Three phases can be distinguished, although each merged almost imperceptibly into the next. In the first and last I believe I gained greater understanding of both our perspectives: my journey into her world forced me to critically examine my own values, but as one year and then two passed, I learned that she, when given a chance, shares these values as well. In the second phase, Colette made a discovery about me: a non-judgmental, interested mother can be very useful.

THE FIRST PHASE

Initially, Colette was suspicious of me, but gradually she began to allow me to spend more time with her. With the increased interaction, I became aware I was really seeing Colette for the first time. I realized she is

—the young matron sitting quietly on a couch, blond hair lifted into a twist at the nape of her neck, wisps falling forward onto her pink cheeks. With hands folded in her lap she gazes distantly through gold-rimmed glasses past the family members milling about her. Their conversation does not interest her.

—the stocky figure careening down the street on her moped wearing a billowing flowered skirt, an orange nylon windbreaker and a crash helmet. The latter all but covers eyes that are fiercely alert for "stupid drivers", as she unceremoniously has dubbed negligent motorists.

—the daughter standing in the kitchen, finger in mouth, eyes mischievous, face dead-pan, as she calculatedly makes an innocent comment, guaranteed to make her father yelp with anger.

—the bare-legged creature cheering Popeye, her attention focused on the television screen, her feet banging on the floor in excitement.

—the wistful woman, eyes filling with tears, who suddenly and enviously has noticed the slim, blossoming body of her 15 year old sister.

In short, Colette was no longer "my retarded daughter", but a fascinating, kaleidoscopic personality.

With the passage of time together, my neutral attitude became more and more genuine. When Colette allowed me to share in her life, I discovered that her aberrant behavior was quite rational if considered from her point of view. Many of her actions stemmed from a need to bolster a self-esteem shaken by experiences encountered when trying to satisfy basic economic, social, and psychological needs. Examples taken from my field notes illustrate how Colette's well-being was frequently undermined as she tried to make a living, seek friends, and fulfill what she saw as her biological destiny as a woman.

Colette worked at the beach restaurant for two years until her father found her a position at a large aerospace corporation where she had employee benefits. While her parents considered Colette fortunate to have the job, she was depressed. As she xeroxed copies hour after hour, she constantly compared herself and her monotonous task with her fellow employees and their more varied opportunities. The contrast disheartened her.

My field notes record a conversation to me over the phone during that period.

"I just want to forget about everything", she said. "I just want to sit and watch TV and forget about the world. I'm sick of what I'm doing. I'm just turning pages and pages and pages. I don't think I'm ever going to get moved into something different."

I sympathized and said it was her choice whether to quit or not, for I knew it was highly unlikely she would ever get promoted.

"I don't want to quit. I need the money. It's just that I want to do different things and I don't think I'm going to get to. I don't like it a bit." She was quiet for a minute.

"I've been pleading with Edgar", she resumed. "I want to stay home and be a housewife."

"We couldn't afford it!" I hear Edgar protest vehemently in the background. Edgar, who had since become employed part-time at the restaurant where Colette used to work, was getting dressed for the night shift.

"You have a good job. Why do you want to quit it?" he demanded.

"It's boring!" exclaimed Colette. "All I do is turn pages. I'll never get a chance to do something else."

Colette's financial problems were further aggravated by a frame of reference inconsistent with her income. She craved the material goods she saw in our family — a microwave oven, pretty furniture, trips to Hawaii, a Bankameri-card — while she had to manage with hand-me-downs and an occasional outing at Disneyland. I reminded her that her father and I struggled for many years, but my words did little to mollify her.

While she found her employment situation discouraging, she was gratified by her many interactions with friends. Colette had met Edgar during high school when her Educationally Retarded class was next to his Educationally Handicapped class. When she left home, Edgar moved in with her. Colette loves to entertain in their apartment, as the following passage from my field notes illustrates.

As the door to Colette's home swung open, my husband and I were greeted by a camera flash and a swarm of laughing young people. Colette pushed her way through the crowd, grabbed me by the hand and led me past the remains of Thanksgiving dinner lined up buffet-style on her long desk. Beaming with culinary pride, she excitedly pointed out the turkey carcass and nearly empty bowls of dressing, mashed potatoes and gravy.

"Hey Colette. Come finish serving the pie", interrupted a neatly attired young man with a crew cut. Heeding his appeal, Colette scurried to the small, oval dining table where Edgar and four eager friends awaited the dispensation. My husband and I accepted small portions as she cut and distributed slices of rather thin but tasty mince pie.

Watching Colette, I mused that pure adrenalin must be keeping her going. Early that morning I had dropped by and learned that Linda, her best friend, and Colette had been up until three a.m. collaborating on two mince pies, a sweet potato dish and stuffing. Because Colette cannot read, Linda had read the recipes while Colette carried out the instructions. Up again at eight a.m., Colette had hustled the bird into the oven and placed donuts and a pot of coffee on the table for friends as she continued her dinner preparations. Later that night I was sure fatigue would set in, but now, serving the pie, she was floating, for she was playing her favorite role, that of housewife and hostess.

"Did you explain to aunt Mary Ann I was sorry I couldn't come to Thanksgiving dinner?" Colette asked as she offered me a squirt of whipped topping for my pie.

"Yes, we did", I assured her.

"I always do my own Thanksgiving dinner", announced Colette, smiling over a tradition she had begun the previous year.

Occasions like Thanksgiving were rare because they were expensive, but her apartment frequently contained young people watching T.V., talking, and drinking cokes — often until the wee hours of the morning. Most were fellow members of a social club for developmentally disabled adults. Colette shared with them the realization that potential friendships are limited to marginal members of society like herself. Other people — even brothers and sisters — may be kind, but they will never permit close sharing. The next section of field notes describes one of the many occasions when Colette revealed she "knows her place".

Colette phoned at 10:30 p.m. to tell me about a trip, she, Edgar, and Linda had made to "Movie World" that day. As she gave details of their adventures, I concluded "Movie World" was Universal Studios.
"We saw where Steve Austin and Jamie Sommers got their operations!" she exclaimed excitedly and then confided that she knew "they didn't really get one".
Colette had such a good time she would like to return.
"I'd like to go back with Melanie and her sweetie", Colette decided, referring to her younger sister and her current beau, "if they wouldn't be offended by us", she added cautiously.

Colette seemed to be able to live with her inferior social position and with the discouraging status of her job, but she vigorously resisted any suggestion that she was incapable of being a mother. The night I introduced my research project, her resentment had poured out. I captured some of it in my notes.

"You're afraid all the time that I'm pregnant — or you're after me to have my tubes tied", she cried. "You feel I'm not capable of taking care of a baby. I *am* capable!"
I reassured her softly that I knew she was capable.
"You said you would disown me if I had a child. You'd never love your own grandchild!" she wailed.
I quietly said that the decision of parenthood was between her and Edgar, and I had nothing to do with that. But if she did have a baby, both she and her child would be welcome in our home.
"Edgar said if I got pregnant, he wouldn't let me have an abortion", she insisted. "I know how to take care of babies. I baby-sit — even tiny ones. And Edgar says I'm good with babies."

In summary, Colette's view of the world was colored by repeated experiences which indicated to her that she was incompetent. Her mother considered her not capable enough to have a baby; her work supervisors found her too deficient to handle the more interesting, better paying tasks, and most of society was off-limits as far as friendship was concerned. While she had openly commented about these problems at one time or another, on only one occasion did she reveal her feelings about her handicap *per se*. I recorded the moment.

Emerging from her apartment, Colette looked very much the modish young office worker with her funky sandals, hosiery, wrap-skirt, and jersey blouse. Her hair was freshly combed and slicked back. Settling herself in the back seat of our car, she sat quietly, subdued.
"Thank you for taking me to the wedding shower", she said softly. Her father said he was happy to do it.
"The present is in this paper bag. I didn't have time to wrap it", she said and paused. Words began to spill out jerkily.

"I wanted to buy a card — I tried to. I went into the store and bought one, but it was the wrong kind."

Choking back tears, she stumbled on.

"I didn't want to go ask the man to read it to me. I wanted to do it myself." She said she made her purchase, rushed home to Edgar and had him read it to her only to discover that although the sentiments were appropriate, the card was written for a man to give to a woman.

"I can't even buy a stupid card!" she cried out in depair.

Silence fell in the car as she struggled to control her emotions, and her father and I, aching with her pain, tried to think of what to say.

When I put all these things together — the low self-esteem and the problems Colette has encountered trying to make her way — I found I had a better appreciation of the toll normalization can take, and I judged her less harshly. When she missed work for a day or two, or even a week, because she was "dizzy", I remembered how bleak she perceived her employment situation to be. When rent money went for rock concert tickets for her and Edgar, I was aware of the affluence she saw in our family. When she talked of wanting to see a doctor because she and Edgar had been unable to conceive, I thought of her as a woman with the same fertility needs as any other female. And when she stayed up all night with her friends, I reminded myself how much emotional support they give her.

Not only had this research experience allowed me to understand Colette's point of view better, it had also caused me to question my formula for her successful survival: "Go to work every day, budget your time carefully, eat right, go to bed early, control your money, and avoid pregnancy". From my new vantage point I recognized how much my rational, middle-class value of self-reliance underscored my prescription. I began to wonder if it might not be too harsh a regimen. There are many kinds of success: the one that was most meaningful for her might well be centered around all-night sessions with friends, a baby or two, and SSI for income. Ten months earlier I would have shuddered at that scenario. With the insight I had gained, I discovered I would be a good deal more accepting if Colette lived in that fashion.[3]

THE SECOND PHASE

The months went by. As the collaboration continued, Colette realized more and more that I was a gratifying resource. Like other researchers who have done field work among the mentally retarded, I became her therapist and advocate (Frank, 1980). She found she could pour out her problems to an uncritical, interested listener, and if she needed help interacting with delivery system professionals, I could be counted on. In addition, as her mother, I could be appealed to, usually successfully, for instrumental help: a run to the drugstore for medicine, a "loan" of money, help with the Christmas baking, or the use of my washing machine and dryer. But as her solicitations and interactions with me increased, I became weary of making notes and exhausted by her seemingly unending problems.

Occasional entries like the following appeared in my notes.

Colette called at 7 pm. I heard her voice and my immediate reaction was the one I gave voice
to: "Oh, no!" She thought something terrible had happened and wanted to know what it was. I
explained I was under great stress at that moment and I just didn't want to have to cope with
her or anyone or anything. I had arrived home from work sick, tired, having had a long day,
and I wanted to go to dinner with my husband and Melanie and relax. Before we could get out
the door, phone calls had held us up, and then, just as we were locking the door, the phone
rang and it was Colette. I felt as if I couldn't stand it if I had to listen to her problems. I kept
trying to ask if I couldn't call her in an hour after I'd had a chance to unwind, but she
explained that wasn't possible. So I had to stand there and try this way and that and another
way to suggest solutions to the problem she presented me with (it involved some extremely
complicated logistics related to my picking up some groceries she had left at a friend's house),
and the whole time I wanted to scream. I felt I couldn't be patient a second longer but
somehow I was.

The problems she struggled with during this period centered around four
issues. A fifth one, that of pregnancy, resolved itself over time. As Edgar and
Colette did not undergo the medical tests necessary to pinpoint the cause of
the infertility having children had apparently receded in importance.

The first issue that remained salient was her job. She disliked everything
about it except the employee benefits. Caught in a quandary, she effectively
postponed making a decision to quit by continuing to malinger. A steady
stream of illnesses and accidents provided excuses for not going to work.
One time she lost her glasses. That day she reported to me, crying, that when
she had gone down to the ocean to "test the water, a big wave knocked (her)
down", and in the process her glasses had disappeared. As she is quite
nearsighted, attendance at work was precluded.

A few days later I recorded the following.

Colette showed up around 5:15 p.m. with strange glasses perched on her nose: heavy tortoise
shell rims in small kewpie shapes, turning up at the corners. She explained that she had just
come from the optometrist who had given her the interim spectacles until her new ones were
ready. I asked if she was able to go to work with them. She answered no, that while the
substitute pair helped, her vision was still too impaired to xerox. She cut off further discussion
by saying it was her problem, not mine.

The second on-going problem was her marital status. She was clearly frustrated over not being married to Edgar. The vicissitudes of their relationship
were rarely, however, topics of conversation with me, for she fiercely
guarded their privacy. The only clues I had were either their behavior when
with me or overheard comments between them when she called me on the
phone. As with most couples, the tenor of these interactions varied. Edgar
could be impatient or solicitous, depending on the situation: when he was
unemployed, he was far more likely to be cross. But even with a regular pay-
check coming in, he could ignore her entreaties when he was absorbed in his
favorite television show. On other occasions, however, he would give her his
full attention. She, in turn, cajoled him, mothered him, and kept dropping
hints within his earshot that she wanted to be his wife.

One day Colette and I were being particularly relaxed at her apartment, and I used the opportunity to discuss the issue.

"Does Edgar really want to marry you?" I asked.

She considered carefully and responded that he *says* he does. "All I know is that he's happy to be here. His mom knows he likes me—loves me. He talks with her about marrying me, and then she tells me some of the things. The only thing he wants is money saved. He wants to get ahead, and that's why we're not married yet." She spoke of Edgar being under a "great deal of pressure" but did not elaborate.

"Do you think Edgar doesn't want to marry me?" she asked. I said I didn't know, that all I knew was that he had been putting it off.

"He wants to get married by a 'free judge' . . . to get it over with", continued Colette. "We can 'renew it' by having a big wedding later. I tell him I don't want that. Would you be upset if I did that?" she asked.

I told her I would be content with anything she wanted.

The third issue was their finances. Although they struggled to understand and control their money, they continued to find it difficult. As they purchased new furniture with cash and enjoyed restaurant dinners along with occasional recreational outings, unpaid bills kept surfacing. Edgar tried to keep track of the medical bills and to fill out Colette's medical insurance forms. It was, however, more than he could handle: one clinic sent a bill to a collection agency, and another clinic threatened to do the same if nearly $500 was not taken care of. In addition, the rent was perpetually behind which required that Colette deal with a grandmother who, although far more lenient than she would have been with any other tenant, still insisted on being paid.

From Colette's perspective, the solution was for her to make more money. She expressed this one day over the phone when I took notes.

Colette continued listing all the things that they need to buy.

"See, these are all the things we're trying to solve. I don't like telling you our business. I feel embarrassed. I feel it's not right nor nothing. We're going through a very difficult, hard stage."

I suggested that perhaps the problem lay in how they manage their money.

Colette answered that her grandmother talks like that. "She doesn't think we know how to handle our money. How else can people enjoy themselves", she demanded, "without staying home, worrying about the stupid rent and blah, blah, blah. I hate telling people about my problems. That's why I'd like to make the amount dad makes."

She again began listing all the things she and Edgar need to buy including a couch that turns into a bed and a new refrigerator. They need to have an income like her father's, she insisted.

The final issue was the ownership of a car. From the beginning of our collaboration, Colette was determined to learn to drive and then to own an automobile. Her parents were almost as firm in their resolve that she not have one. We felt she could not afford one and that her judgment as a driver would be inadequate. She was not to be deterred. After convincing the Department of Rehabilitation to fund a tutor to teach her the vehicle code, she passed the exam. The Department of Rehabilitation was again solicited, this time to underwrite driver training. The agency complied, and Colette sailed through the driving test. Badgering us to lend her the money for a car began in earnest as that point. Our resolve weakening, we announced that her debts must be cleared up first.

Meanwhile, she found a temporary means of obtaining an automobile. Her ingenuity was first revealed in a phone conversation.

> Colette returned my phone call and cheerfully said she knew why I was calling: it was to set a time when I could help Edgar with the medical bills, as he had requested. She then covered the phone with her hand, and I could hear a muffled, rather heated, exchange. Colette finally resumed talking to me. Edgar had agreed it was okay to tell me about the car, she said. They had rented one.
>
> I was careful to be neutral as I said, "Oh?" and she cooed about how beautiful it was. We agreed I could come right then to work with Edgar, and I could see it.
>
> I arrived shortly and was taken into the tiny garage to see the prize, a new white Toyota-Corolla, the kind she had always dreamed of owning. She insisted I sit in the driver's seat and inspect the interior. I did so and noticed popcorn scattered over the floor area. Colette explained that the night before they had gone with friends to a drive-in movie and had had a "super" time.

As these problems engulfed both Colette and me, I was incapable of attaining, much less sustaining, any perspective as far as our relationship was concerned. Only now, as I review the field notes of that period, do I realize that what we both went through was necessary. She needed to be let alone to work things out for herself, and my pulling back into a detached observer's stance gave her that opportunity. Yet, almost paradoxically, she needed me to be involved — to listen to her woes, to act as an intermediary with medical clinic bookkeepers when she felt overwhelmed, and to provide assistance like giving her a lift home from the supermarket with groceries because it was raining, or slipping some money into her purse when her billfold was stolen. Actually, in juggling these two demands of being neutral yet ready to help I was doing little more than what Galinsky (1981) reports is required of any parent whose child is departing from home. She found that the more successful parents had a "dual empathy", a "seeing the world through one's own and one's children's eyes, while being cognizant they are two separate visions". It appears that parents need to develop much the same skills as ethnographers.

THE THIRD PHASE

The problems that plagued Colette were gradually resolved in the final period of our collaboration. First, she was discharged from the xeroxing position. She was now free to resume part-time employment at the beach restaurant working alongside Edgar. There, in contrast to repetitious copy-making, her duties are varied, and she feels she is a valued employee. Not surprisingly, illnesses and accidents have ceased to trouble her.

Second, with two incomes coming in (both she and Edgar were soon moved into full-time employee status), the two young people paid off their medical bills. Keeping his word, her father loaned her the money for a car and helped her pick it out. It was not a new Toyota-Corolla, but Colette proved flexible.

Third, Colette and Edgar have married. I do not know what convinced Edgar it was the right thing to do, but, becoming consistently more affectionate toward Colette, he suddenly announced he wanted a big wedding, entered into the planning enthusiastically, and one sunny afternoon two years and four months after Colette and I had begun our project, he took a happy but very stage-frightened Colette as his wife.

The minister gave me a copy of the notes he used when speaking before the over 100 assembled guests. In one section of the ceremony, drawing on pre-nuptual conversations he had had with the couple, he described the bride and groom.

Edgar—child of the beach, lover of rock and roll, watcher of movies, especially the martial arts. Liker of people, T.V., and baseball. Not afraid to work. Edgar is Colette's eyes, her lover, her precious. Easily upset, easy to forgive. A man who lives and sees life simply, who sees his life only with Colette.

   Colette—laughing and giggling at life, lover of swimming and riding horses. Edgar's lover. She likes to go places, especially with Edgar. Proud of learning to live alone, she says, the "hard way". She treasures her freedom but wishes she could stay home more to cook and sew. Tender and understanding. Edgar says, "She makes me feel so good".

I have gained new insights as these issues have been resolved. Because Colette has attained two very normalizing statuses, those of wife and car owner, and because she has a job where her very real contribution is recognized by both supervisors and fellow employees, her self-esteem has markedly improved. Feeling better about herself, her response to both her father and me is different. Now she is quite willing to accept bookkeeping help from him, something she never permitted as long as she felt she had to prove herself; with their money, her father keeps track of and pays their medical and automotive bills. At the same time, the frequency of her phone calls to me has decreased dramatically, and we see each other only a little more often than we did before the study began. The tenor of the interactions is quite different, however. She and Edgar come to dinner, after Edgar has approved the menu, or they borrow our camping gear for a week-end in the mountains, or Colette comes by to bring her father money for medical and car expenses.

The relationship is much like that of any parent with their married daughter who lives nearby, except that we provide more instrumental help. I was far more of a resource for Colette than I am now for my son as he leaves home, and I am convinced that throughout Colette's life, her well-being in great measure will depend on her knowing there is a parent or sibling who cares and is available should she need help. A responsive family member provides a stability as well as a social-emotional gratification unlike that of any delivery system arrangement, no matter how enlightened or well-meaning that arrangement may be (Zetlin, Turner, and Winik, in press).

Her outcome is not the scenario I was prepared to accept toward the end of the first phase of the research. Today Colette only rarely enjoys all-night sessions with friends, does not have a child, and is not collecting SSI. Instead, she and Edgar, like the rest of us, put in their work week, scramble to get the laundry and cleaning done and the groceries purchased on their days off, and hope that they have time to get away for a few days now and then. The middle class notion of self-reliance that I had earlier accepted as too demanding for Colette appears to have been thoroughly adopted not only by her but also by her husband.

Colette's and my relationship underwent a significant transformation during the time covered in this account. By attempting to be more objective I gained many valuable insights into both my daughter and myself. Perhaps there is a lesson for others as well.

NOTES

1. I have been a Staff Research Associate at the Socio-Behavioral Group of the Mental Retardation Research Center, University of California at Los Angeles, since 1979. This study was part of a larger investigation of personal and social adjustment of retarded persons living in community settings directed by R. Gallimore, J. Turner, and A. Zetlin. Without the help and encouragement of these individuals, as well as that of my co-workers Grace Davis, Joe Graffam, Jean Heriot, Frank Marlowe, Doug Valpey, and Lesley Winik, this research would not have been possible.
2. Akemi Kikumura, when recording the life history of her Issei mother, encountered a similar phenomenon. The older woman tended to describe the years after Akemi was born "with an economy of detail" because she assumed Akemi remembered the events as well as, or possibly even better than, she (Kikumura, 1981).
3. Much of the preceding material appeared in Kaufman (1980).

REFERENCES

Edgerton, R.
  1982 The cloak of competence. Berkeley: University of California Press.
Frank, G.
  1980 Intervention: ethics and objectivity in participant observation with the mildly retarded. (Working Paper No. 17). Socio-Behavioral Group, Mental Retardation Research Center, School of Medicine, University of California, Los Angeles.
Galinsky, E.
  1981 Between generations: the six stages of parenthood. New York: Quandrangle/The New York Times Book Company, Inc.
Kaufman, S. Z.
  1980 A mentally retarded daugther educates her mother. Exceptional Parent, 10 (6): 17–22.
Kikumura, A.
  1981 Through harsh winters: The life of a Japanese immigrant woman. Novato, California: Chandler and Sharp Publishers, Inc.

Langness, L. and Frank, G.
    1981 *Lives: An anthropological approach to biography*. Novato, California: Chandler and
        Sharp Publishers, Inc.
Turner, J.
    1980 Yes I am human: Autobiography of a "retarded career". *Journal of Community
        Psychology, 8*: 3—8.
Zetlin, A., Turner, J. and Winik, L.
    in press. Socialization effects on the adult adaptation of mildly retarded persons living in
        the community. *In* S. Landesman-Dwyer and P. Vietze, (eds.), *The impact of
        residential settings on behavior*. Baltimore: University Park Press.

PAUL KOEGEL

YOU ARE WHAT YOU DRINK: EVIDENCE OF SOCIALIZED INCOMPETENCE IN THE LIFE OF A MILDLY RETARDED ADULT

The last two decades have been characterized by a growing appreciation of the ways in which socio-cultural factors influence the phenomenon of mental retardation. Whereas we once viewed mental retardation solely through biomedical and psychological perspectives and thus restricted our attention to individuals and their symptoms, we now more readily acknowledge the extent to which mental retardation is socially defined and the very strong impact which the social world surrounding an individual exerts on his or her life course. This in turn has made us realize that answers to questions such as "Who eventually is identified as retarded?" and "What will their lives be like?" are neither fixed nor the exclusive function of individual capability. Who gets labeled, and what happens to them once they are labeled, is very much tied to the social, cultural, and economic contexts in which they find themselves. As a result, we have come to accept that a full appreciation of mental retardation demands the understandings which a socio-cultural perspective can yield.

In spite of this realization, it is often difficult for researchers and lay people alike to push aside the blinders imposed on them by the clinical/ medical model which has traditionally prevailed. When faced with a person exhibiting behavior which leads us to suspect that he or she is retarded, that behavior, whatever its form, is believed to reflect some sort of deficit in the physiological or cognitive machinery which allows non-retarded individuals to perform as fully functioning members of our society. However much we pay lip service to the influence of socio-cultural factors, we *do* primarily see mental retardation as a biomedical phenomenon and *do*, as a result, tend to attribute incompetent behavior exclusively to physiological causes.

An unfortunate consequence of this tendency is that we rarely consider the possibility that at least some of the incompetent behavior exhibited by mentally retarded individuals may be the result of experiential, and even environmental, rather than constitutional, factors. However important organic and cognitive limitations may be in inhibiting intellectual ability and adaptive potential, the fact remains that mentally retarded people, like all of us, are as much a product of how they are raised as they are of the constraints with which they are born. It thus stands to reason that the socialization experiences they undergo may play a significant role in influencing the competence they ultimately display. Given this, any number of realities linked to the socialization process — the attitudes of those around them as to what they can and cannot do, the experiences they are allowed to have and those they are discouraged from having, the different arenas of

47

L. L. Langness and H. G. Levine (eds.), Culture and Retardation, 47—63.
© *1986 by D. Reidel Publishing Company.*

social learning in which they have opportunities to participate, the kinds of information to which they exposed — all become as relevant to a consideration of their developing competence as the cognitive factors which have preoccupied us for so long.

This chapter explores the notion that at least some of the non-normative behaviors exhibited by mentally retarded individuals are artifacts of a unique process of socialization which somehow manages to create incompetence where it need not exist. It begins by examining on a conceptual level the evidence which might lead us to suspect the existence of such a process. But it quickly moves on to a more empirical level, looking closely at the life of one mildly retarded adult for evidence of this process in operation. In portraying how attitudes, expectations, and the structuring of opportunity on the part of this individual's family have profoundly influenced his social competence, it ultimately suggests the significance of this avenue of inquiry and hopefully lays the groundwork for further research along these lines.

WHY SOCIALIZATION?

Two questions immediately come to mind in considering the relationship between socialization and the competence of mentally retarded individuals: (1) Why should we suspect that socialization might affect the competence of mentally retarded individuals?, and (2) How might a unique and continuing socialization experience be translated into consequences for the competence of these individuals. Let us begin with the first.

As much as we shy away from calling mental retardation "deviance", perhaps because deviance for some people (Farber, 1968) implies an intentional flouting of society's norms, deviance theory stands as an excellent starting point for the answer to the first question. Over the last twenty years, the emphasis within deviance theory has shifted from a preoccupation with the issue of what *causes* people to commit deviant acts to a concern with the social process which is set into motion once individuals are recognized as being "deviant" (Becker, 1963; Filstead, 1972; Rubington and Weinberg, 1973). As a result of this concern, attention has been focused on the post-labeling experiences of a wide variety of individuals — mental patients (Goffman, 1959; Scheff, 1966), heroin addicts (Ray, 1964), petty thieves (Cameron, 1973), and male hustlers (Reiss, 1964) to name but a few — and a paradigm of the social process which labeling sets into motion has emerged. Once defined as a deviant by his social audience, it seems, an individual's world undergoes radical changes. Assumptions as to who he is and what can be expected of him are suddenly revised. The social opportunities available to him are suddenly realigned. The groups with which he is pressured to identify are altered, and the substance of his interactions with others modified. Given the pervasive quality of these social realignments and altered expectations, their subtle and not so subtle effects on the individual's existence, and the reflexive nature of self-concept in general, the labeled individual eventually begins to define himself as others define him and act as others expect him to act. Ultimately, in other words, the individual has been socialized into a socially constructed role. And it is this role, which finds its substance not in the deviant act itself but in the configuration of attitudes, beliefs, and values held by the social audience regarding the person who committed it, which determines much of his future behavior.

Deviance theory, then, leads us to the conclusion that the socialization experiences which disabled individuals undergo may be as limiting as their handicap itself. But it is not only on the basis of theory that we might suspect a relationship between socialization and the incompetence of the retarded. Actual cases, presented in both popular and academic forums, similarly point to the salient role which socialization can potentially play in fostering helplessness and dependency. "Larry", for instance, a television dramatiza-tion, depicted the experiences of a young, institutionalized and apparently severely retarded man who was later discovered to possess normal intel-ligence. In spite of his innate intelligence, Larry's lack of training in even the fundamentals of social existence, as well as his complete and overwhelming naivete regarding social relations and transactions, indeed rendered him "retarded". Equally relevant is the case documented by Edgerton (1975) of a man whom he calls John Millon, who was labeled mentally retarded at the age of four but discovered at the age of 18 to have on I.Q. of 102. Despite his average intelligence and the absence, in his case, of prolonged institu-tionalization, this young man found himself unprepared for an independent, self-sufficient way of life. His pattern of being locked into roles of depend-ency and his basic lack of experience made it difficult for him to adjust to life as a "normal" person, and actually led him to confess that "It was much ea-sier to be retarded" (Edgerton, this volume). Similarly, Turner (1980) offers the story of Doug Valpey, a man who was considered by himself and others to be retarded until he reached the age of 35, at which time a battery of tests revealed him to be a well-adjusted individual with average intelligence. As was the case with Larry and John, there was much about Doug which made him *seem* retarded. It was only after a protracted period of time that a new persona, consistent with his new self-image as a non-retarded individual, began to emerge (Turner, 1981).

A very clear message emerges from each of these cases: individuals of normal measured intelligence who are raised as if they are mentally retarded find themselves ill-prepared to cope with the demands of everyday existence and the mechanics of social interaction. From this realization, it is but a small step to the idea that factors relating to their socialization experiences may similarly limit the potential of mentally retarded individuals themselves. It may be case that mislabeled individuals can, if given the chance, learn to fill a normal social role, whereas "bona fide" mentally retarded individuals cannot. But even so, cases such as these distinctly point to the possibility that at least some of the incompetent behavior which retarded individuals exhibit may be a result of the way in which they are raised.

The issue of *how* this process actually works is far more complicated than the question of why we might suspect it exists. The attitudes we hold regarding mental retardation, however, stand as crucial starting points in figuring out how socialization for incompetence actually takes place. There are, of course, as many attitudes toward mental retardation as there are people, and exceptions will exist to any generalizations I may make. But even so, certain common beliefs, however implicit, do seem to underlie the way in which we deal with retardation in mainstream Anglo society. We tend to believe, for instance, that the retarded — even the mildly retarded — remain children, in a sense, throughout their lives; that they never quite reach adulthood. We also tend to assume that they together form a relatively homogeneous group — that all retarded individuals, in other words, are capable and incapable of doing the same things. Likewise, we tend to hold the notion that the incompetence which results from their disability is pervasive and all-encompassing, necessarily affecting all that they do. And we are convinced, somehow, that they, as handicapped individuals, are more different from us than they are alike, and must thus be dealt with according to a separate set of rules and practices.

The importance of these attitudes lies in the fact that they influence, even determine, the substance of our interactions with retarded individuals and the nature of the experiences we allow them to have. We tend to talk down to them, for instance, and treat them as if they were children regardless of their age. We direct their behavior, leaving them little room in which to exercise initiative. We rescue them at the merest hint of a problem. We do for them, rather than teach them to do for themselves. We regulate their lives, rather than encouraging them to become self-sufficient and autonomous. We nervously shield them from situations which involve risk. We even more nervously approach the idea of their engaging in "adult" activities such as sex, and question the wisdom of allowing them to fool with socially accepted "vices" which we ourselves enjoy. We somehow assume that there are things which they will never be able to do or are better off not doing — driving a car, for instance, or marrying — and organize their activities in a way which is consistent with these assumptions. We shy away from making certain demands of them. We rarely expect them to take responsibility for themselves and tend not to allow them to make the major and minor decisions which affect their existence. We carefully choose the kinds of information available to them so as not to tease them with the thought of things we feel they will never have. We convince them, as best we can, that it is truly better for them to lead circumscribed lives. And we restrict, however inadvertently, the nature of their participation in social circles of non-retarded individuals.

In the end, these practices foster incompetence in two ways. The first of these has to do with self-perception and the way it influences behavior. Like all of us, retarded people are to a large degree dependent on others for a sense of who they are and what they are capable of doing. Like us, their self-concept (Blumer, 1969; Mead, 1940), or perhaps more precisely, their self-understanding (Damon and Hart, 1982), evolves out of the evaluations of their behavior and abilities which are implicit in the interactions they have with others. Regardless of their potential ability, retarded individuals (as well as those who are only thought to be retarded, as we have seen) tend to receive a rather uniform set of direct and subtle messages from the inter-actions in which they are typically involved — messages to the effect that they are helpless, dependent, child-like, and incapable of such things as exercising initiative, assuming responsibility for themselves, or mastering any number of tasks.

The second way in which the above practices serve to foster incompetence has to do with what we give the mentally handicapped the chance to learn. As has already been noted, our tendency is to think of the incompetence of mentally handicapped individuals — even the mildly handicapped — as being all-encompassing. We don't see their handicap as something which will significantly affect them only in certain ways, such as in their performance in school, or the occupations available to them, or the length of time it takes for them to master tasks, or even their ability to appreciate higher order levels of humor. Rather, we start by assuming that the fact of their retardation will affect *everything* they do. In the process, we sometimes allow the attitudes, assumptions, and expectations which are proper and appropriate in areas where a normative level of competence will never be attained by the retarded to spill over into areas where a more normative level of competence *is* achievable. We assume, for instance, that they will never be able to ride a bicycle, or cook for themselves, or handle sharp knives, or ride the bus. As a result, we deny them the opportunity to learn such things through the very processes by which we all learn them — by trying, failing, learning from our mistakes, and practicing. On top of this, we hold attitudes and engage in social practices which tend to isolate them, at least from their non-retarded peers. As a result, we also end up reducing their opportunities to learn though interaction and experience, in the way their normal counterparts do, the knowledge, attitudes and subtle nuances of behavior associated with people their age.

My argument then, is that a number of factors which stem as much from the attitudes we hold about mental retardation as the disability of mental retardation itself — factors such as the messages the retarded receive about how they should behave and what they are capable of, their reduced oppor-tunities to learn behavior which they may in fact be capable of learning, their lack of exposure to certain kinds of information and interaction — together operate to restrict their potential and, what is more, actually produce in-competence where it need not exist.

METHODOLOGICAL CONSIDERATIONS

In 1976, the Socio-Behavioral Group of the UCLA Mental Retardation Research Center initiated a project which sought to closely examine the everyday lives of 48 mildly retarded adults living in their communities. A primary objective of this project was simply to reach an understanding of the life-styles of mildly retarded adults and to document the process of their adaptation to community life. But our goal was also to determine the ways in which various people, places, and practices either facilitate or hinder their ability to lead more independent and self-sufficient lives. Success in reaching these goals, we hoped, would provide both a richer understanding of the needs, hopes, values, problems, and abilities of the mildly retarded and a better sense of how the "normalization principle" was being implemented in practice, as opposed to theory.

Our strategy in attempting to understand these mildly retarded and the methodology we employed has been described elsewhere (Edgerton and Langness, 1978).

In what follows, I focus on one of the 48 individuals in our sample — John Hamlin[1] — as an example of how the socialization experiences which mildly retarded individuals undergo can create incompetence where it need not exist. Recognizing that I cannot, within this chapter, do justice to John's life as a whole, I examine one incident in detail, John's first experience with alcohol, which typifies certain features of his socialization. The ultimate effect of this incident on John's competence, I realize, might be dismissed by some as inconsequential in the larger scheme of his life. The importance of this incident, however, lies in the fact that it is characteristic of the experiences of many mentally retarded individuals. It clearly shows how the beliefs of socialization agents regarding what is right, proper, and possible for their retarded charges can dramatically affect both their opportunities for learning and their self-understanding.

JOHN AND HIS FAMILY

Short and solidly built, John is a pleasant looking man whose dramatically receding hairline and dark facial hair lend the impression that he is somewhat older than his 25 years. Marring his otherwise normal physiognomy and build are the droopy lids which hang low over John's eyes, giving his other-wise bright and animated countenance a slightly vacant quality. This stig-matizing feature, which resulted from an infection following an operation, is a central concern of John's. He once confessed (after observing himself on videotape) that he believed his lids led others to imagine that he is in danger of falling asleep.

Best characterized as a sociable person, John is an individual who in-tensely enjoys interaction with other people, whether it be ordinary social conversation or the chance to entertain with his guitar, auto harp and pleasant voice. Quick to laugh, chat, sing, dance, tell or appreciate a joke, John is equally amenable to serious conversation and will, if asked or if troubled, thoughtfully contemplate the myriad events of his own life, expressing his feelings in an articulate and often provocative manner. His high level of communicative competence is paralleled by his general bearing and manners. Always the gentleman, John would no more think of sitting down at the dinner table without a napkin on his lap than he would of stepping outside without his clothes.

Despite the social talents he does indeed possess, John manages to be a master of the *faux pas*, more often than not in social settings where he is feeling comfortable and expansive, such as gatherings of family and family friends. Outwardly manifesting signs that he would love nothing more than to be "one of the gang", he tends, much to the amusement of his audience, to deliver baffling quips with confusing sexual innuendos (sex being a subject about which he remains painfully naive), to introduce topics that might better be left alone, and to reveal more of himself than he would in less familiar settings where he is more guarded, all of which draw attention to him as an "incompetent" individual. Further, the anxiety he betrays in new situations, an anxiety that inhibits the skills he indeed possesses, is surprising. While completely at ease in any restaurant, amusement park or any number of public places he has frequented in the past, when faced with the unfamiliarity of a recreation complex where we spent a Saturday, John, whose amazing sense of direction can ordinarily take him anywhere he desires, was suddenly sure than if forced to find and enter by himself the locker room not fifty yards away, he would be unable to locate the bathroom within it. In the locker room as well, John's anxiety, his overt concern over proper comportment, and his ill-concealed shock at realizing that men showered without swim suits in the communal shower room masked his usual competence, and called attention to himself.

John is presently employed part-time in the factory of a family friend, a job requiring a fair share of responsibility as well as four hours of daily travel on public transportation involving different buses. He lives at home with his parents in a spacious house. Neither John nor his parents see any change in his living status within the near future. John's brief flirtation with the idea was not rejected or criticized by Mr. and Mrs. Hamlin but they did point out that it would be rather difficult for him to move into an apartment with a friend on a salary of a mere sixty dollars a week. Without encouragement, John soon lost interest in the idea.

Despite his parents' despair over what they see as his ignorance concerning the value of money, John's skills are such that he could, with some coaching and supervision, live on his own. Still, he remains at home, spending an inordinate amount of time alone, entertaining himself with the large number of material possessions that his parents' wealth has enabled him to accumulate. His solitary pattern is broken occasionally by a Saturday expedition with the few friends with whom he has kept in contact from his days in a private school for developmentally delayed individuals and the transitional workshop at which he later worked for a year.

I first met John at a gathering of a leisure club catering specifically to mildly mentally retarded adults to which he then belonged. For two years, I visited John on a weekly to bi-weekly basis, spending hours with him at various sites filled with in-depth conversation.

JOHN'S FIRST EXPERIENCE WITH ALCOHOL

Of the many stories in the Hamlin family repertoire, there is one which remains particularly alive in the minds of all of those who had been involved. It was recounted to me by each of the participants on separate occasions — John, his mother, his father, his brother, and a family friend — each unaware that another had already reported the event. Indeed, so vivid was this story in their minds that each shared it with me more than once, usually as some current happening brought it to mind.

From the four similar accounts, the following picture emerges. John, uncomfortable at restaurants unless familiar with the menu and aware of what he can order in advance, often chose to remain at home on occasions when his parents and brother explored new restaurants. On one such occasion, when he was about 21, the Hamlins returned to the house with friends only to find John sitting in his "dad's chair" with his feet propped up on the coffee table, a drink in his hand. Overtly unconcerned, his dad affably asked him what he was drinking and learned that it was a scotch and seven-up. Interested in what was to him a novel combination, Ed indicated that he was going to have to try that, but in the meanwhile wondered aloud if John had ever tried bourbon and water. No? Why then he would have to try one of those . . . .

And so the evening proceeded. Joined by Dan and Dick, a family friend, Ed urged John to explore a smorgasbord of drinks which he prepared on the spot. By the end of the evening, all participants were more than slightly inebriated. John, ever so proud to be "drinking with the men", had attacked with great gusto whatever had been placed in front of him. But since he had less practice than the others in the art of swilling down large quantities of alcohol, his method of proving himself backfired. Before long, he was completely intoxicated and proceeded to be sick. In John's words, "I was so sick I couldn't stand it. I was out on the balcony — my parents took me out there 'cause I couldn't sleep. I was climbing the walls. And they were holding me out there and I was throwing up down the embankment. I was so sick I had a hangover for three days." Dan confirmed. "He was the human vomit bazooka! Boy, we were holding him like a bazooka. Holding his feet and propping him against the railing, letting him barf right over the hill." Lee

confessed that she has since worried that they might have killed John, such
was the amount he had consumed, and ruefully recalled how he had been
unable to get out of bed for two days straight, having only enough energy to
turn his head to the side to fill the pail she had strategically placed by his
side. Ed, however, calmly pointed to the efficacy of what he refers to as his
"cure": "You go into a restaurant and I'll have a scotch and water and Dan
will have a scotch and water and John will order a glass of milk. And he's not
embarassed about asking for it." John has indeed "learned his lesson". He
consistently refuses any offers of alcohol and invokes the above story if
pressed for an explanation. "I finally found that it didn't pay to drink", he
said. "Now it's just straight apple juice or soft drinks but nothin' more than
that".

Interestingly, Ed and Lee indicated that "the same thing" had been done to
Dan when he was young, and Dan himself wryly admitted that "the first time
I ever got drunk, Dad got me drunk". Having observed Dan with a drink in
his hand on many social occasions, I commented to the Hamlins that it
seemed to me that Dan had overcome the "cure". At that, Ed admitted that
the procedure he had followed with John was different:

When Dan was younger he was playing a lot of jobs. At age sixteen people were pushing
drinks toward him and he had to drive home. All I wanted Dan to do was . . . I just said to
him, "Listen, do you know what your capacity is?" He said, "No". And I said, "Some night I
think you ought to find out so that if you're playing at this part somewhere and you gotta
drive, you know what you can handle". Well, he came home one night when I was working and
he ups and says, "Let's find out what my capacity is". So we sat down and drank. After about
the fourth drink he said, "I don't feel like my feet are touching the floor". I said, "O.K. Then I'd
stop at three". It wasn't for the same purpose. I wasn't trying to get him drunk. I was just trying
to get him to find out what he could handle.

In fact, then, two different approaches had been applied to similar episodes
in the lives of John and Dan. The Hamlins eventually acknowledged this but
felt strongly that their different reactions were necessary and proper. They
argued that Dan's ability to reason facilitated and even demanded an intellectual, logical approach while John's childhood had taught them that he had
to be "hit over the head" — "the old story of getting the attention of the
mule". Further, they said, Dan's sense of responsibility meant that he had an
equal interest in controlling his intake of alcohol. Ed's approach with Dan
was thus, "Hey. I'm not gonna watch you 24 hours a day. I don't care what
you do. Just know what you can handle", an approach he did not feel was
applicable to John.

Dan recognized that his education had been designed to teach him his
"limit" while John's was calculated to produce a real aversion to alcohol and
offered the following assessment.

Well they (his parents) didn't . . . I don't think they really . . . I think John surprised them with
his drinking. You know, John would see me come in from school or whatever and pour myself

a shot or a beer or something and he was curious about it so he started sneaking it. And I don't think my parents were ready to consider the fact that he might think that this was the social thing to do. There seemed to be something grown up about it, something important about it. So John would say, "Hey man. I'm gonna pour myself a shot", and my dad would say, "Oh no your aren't! It's two in the afternoon", or whatever. You know, I think he surprised them with his desire to drink. They had never really considered that an option or a threat — the fact that not only could he go 'bye-bye' into T.V. land but that he could pollute himself at the same time and enjoy it twice as much. When you can't do anything and you've got nothing to do, it sure is a lot more fun to be living up to the limit of your ability. So I think he surprised them and it became a threat. If he became an alcoholic on top of everything else, what could they do to salvage him at all, you know? They did handle it a lot different and I think maybe they did the right thing.

Taken by itself, the incident in which John was taught that drinking was not to be a part of his world clearly reveals basic attitudes that have influenced the continuing process of his socialization. In juxtaposing this incident against the handling of the same "problem" in Dan's life, these attitudes become all the more visible. It was accepted, we've seen, that Dan, at age 16, would be drinking. This was understood to be part of maturing, of beginning to travel within certain social circles. The Hamlins, as his parents, felt the obligation to exert their influence to see that he handled alcohol sensibly. It was shocking, though, that at 21 John should begin experimenting with alcohol despite the fact that he too was reaching typically adult milestones — he had finished school for instance, and was responsibly employed. Despite the emphasis placed on treating John as an adult and on raising their sons on the basis of similar principles, points which the Hamlins have often stressed, this incident reveals that the reality of the situation has at times fallen short of the ideal. Certainly in this instance, and in myriad others, John was assumed to be a child.

Interwoven with this subtle acceptance of John as "child", however, is the issue of John's disability and how the Hamlins appreciate it as structuring John's capabilities. The Hamlins have long accepted John as being mildly brain damaged. They believe that John is lacking part of the neurological "circuitry" necessary for him to make certain judgments. They invoke this explanation, however, with no real consistency and seem to be confused as to what John can and cannot learn. Ed, for instance, will suggest in one breath that John's amorality in the early stages of his childhood was a function of the fact that "part of the circuitry that's missing (in John and people like him) has to do with moral sense", thereby offering a biological basis for John's behavior. He will, in the next breath though, point out that John's been "so indoctrinated into moral attitudes that he's overmoral to the point, you know, where you begin to worry about it", a statement implying that John indeed had or developed the full capacity to be socialized into a set of moral principles. John's eventual internalization of a highly developed moral code has not altered, in the minds of the Hamlins, the validity of their assumption that John's ability to make moral judgments is seriously impaired.

While the drinking incident affords one such example of the operation of these attitudes, countless others exist. Another simple example may be seen in a comment made by Lee to John as the two of us prepared to fix ourselves a sandwich after the movies. As John withdrew a cold roast from the refrigerator at Lee's directive, he queried, "How's this thing gonna get sliced?" "By asking your father or Paul to do it!" was Lee's quick reply. Despite the fact that John is quite agile and coordinated, Lee's image of him as a child led her to assume that John shouldn't be "fooling around" with sharp knives.

Yet another example is John's first experience with smoking. Ed and Dan both smoke pipes. When John, who in Lee's words "wanted to be one of the group", decided that he too was ready to indulge, Ed took the following approach: "I gave him a pipe that was just a burner. It was so hot you couldn't stand it. And John lit up and smoked with the rest of us and I could see his tongue was blistering. It's been sitting in his room and he hasn't touched it since." Again, we see the assumption that John should not be treated as "one of the men" but rather as a child. The relatively harmless nature of smoking a pipe highlights this point even further.

These and similar incidents point to the existence of a *spill-over effect* — the differential application of rules, in other words, in areas that need not be affected by John's presumed disabilities but that *are* ultimately affected as a result of the attitudes and assumptions organized around the generalized perception of John as a handicapped individual.

The Hamlins retain a general image of John as a child. Because they suspect that John's failure to develop competence in hazy arenas such as "morality" and "good judgment" on "schedule" has meant that he is incapable of fully developing in such areas (despite evidence that they recognize to the contrary), they've assumed that John must be *conditioned*. In this incident it was assumed for one or both of the above reasons that John would be unable to handle the responsibility involved in drinking sensibly, that he would fail to understand the social context of drinking, that he would be unable to drink in socially acceptable amounts, and that he would abuse alcohol.

The overwhelming consequence of being conditioned in this way is that John has been denied the chance to learn something that is indeed learned. No one is born with an understanding of appropriate drinking behavior; such behavior is culturally determined and transmitted (MacAndrew and Edgerton, 1969). Some of us recall that this learning process involves drinking too much and making a fool of oneself, even becoming ill. Further, it involves feeling secure with one's adult status and not feeling the necessity of drinking to prove oneself. Yet further, it involves practice within social settings and the resulting knowledge of not only what one can handle but what is appropriate. Dan himself, despite the responsibility the Hamlins assumed he possessed, can vividly remember the taste of whiskey sours coming out of his nose and "praying over the porcelain idol after discovering Tequila Gold".

Dan was taught that such discomfort will result from the *abuse* of alcohol; John was taught the lesson that paralyzing illness will be the result of *any* experience he may have with alcohol.

This is not to say the lesson will be enduring. The time may come when John again asserts his right to a drink and at such time the reaction may well be different and far more favorable. But even so, damage has been done in that John has lost time. At the age of 30, perhaps, he will be going through the process that many of his age have completed a decade past, this "retarded" social behavior providing further validation of his incompetent label. This evidence of incompetence, however, relates in no direct way to his disability. Rather, it is an artifact of the socially constructed reality that has emerged from his placement in a "disabled role".

Equally important is the impact this has on how John views himself, on how others view him and on the extent to which John can participate in social circles appropriate for his age.

Take the issue of how John defines himself, for instance. While John insists that he is not bothered by his abstinence, and has made no overt comments expressing a conscious feeling that he has been relegated to the role of child, he offers evidence in more subtle ways that the implicit message encoded in this situation has not been lost on him. He gives every indication that he is aware that drinking and smoking are very "adult" behaviors, ones, indeed, which those around him heavily prize. The stories he has told highlighting the expertise of his adult male role models in such pursuits — the ability of Dick to consume unrivaled quantities of scotch; a fishing trip during which Ed, Dick, and Dan constructed a huge pyramid out of the scores of beer cans the three men had emptied; the proud exhibition of his father's pipe collection; the descriptions of his brother's experiences in bars — all bear witness to this. Since he also realizes that he is consistently discouraged from engaging in such activities, he cannot help but absorb, even if only subconsciously, the idea that he is neither being treated as an adult nor expected to fill an adult role. This incident alone, of course, is not solely responsible for his understanding of himself as something less than an adult. In fact, it is only one of many which continually reinforce this idea.

John's image of himself as one who hasn't truly reached adult status has an impact on how he ultimately behaves: because he doesn't see himself as an adult, he doesn't always see the wisdom, the need, or the appropriateness of acting like an adult. Obvious examples of this abound, such as his assumption that he is dependent on his parents for help in such things as inserting a rectal thermometer. But equally compelling are more subtle ones, such as his basic acceptance of his parents' unquestioned right to make decisions for him. When Ed and Lee restricted him from seeing a woman whom he had dated on numerous occasions but of whom they disapproved, for instance, John protested but acquiesced. Months later, when his desire to see this woman was rekindled, his strategy become one of convincing his parents that she was a suitable companion for him. He conceded, however, that in the event of his failing to reach his stated goal, he would have no recourse but to bow to his parents' wishes. He rejected wholeheartedly the alternative of insisting that he, as an adult, should be allowed to exert autonomy and make his own decisions — indeed, the idea never occurred to him. Rather, he accepted, and continues to accept, that his parents are better able to judge what is best for him, whether he agrees or disagrees.

In the same way that John's practice of abstinence contributes to the way he sees himself, it affects the way others see him. John's abstinence, and even more importantly, the vivid story he tells to explain his abstinence, communicates that he is someone who is "special", and who thus warrants "special treatment": an older person who is nevertheless not really an adult. This is not to say that this is the *only* aspect of John's behavior which imparts this message. Were John to suddenly begin drinking, he would not instantaneously be viewed and treated by others as an ordinary adult. It is to say, however, that John's abstinence and the rationale he offers for it do represent elements in a complex constellation of indicators which direct others to think of him differently, and to act toward him accordingly. Each of these elements in and of themselves may seem minor. But together they coalesce into a compelling statement which profoundly alters the nature of John's interactions with others.

John's view of himself and the way he is viewed by others carries with it one further set of consequences: they end up curtailing his participation in normal social circles and restricting his opportunities to learn, through interaction and experience, the kinds of behavior which are appropriate to one of his chronological years. Because John's sense of himself as an adult is less than complete, first of all, and because he does not engage in certain activities that typically accompany adult social interaction (such as drinking), there is a tendency for him to *absent himself* from such social groupings, despite his love of social activity. At no time did this become more clear than on the occasion of his 25th birthday. In honor of this milestone, Ed and Lee invited a small group of people to the house for an informal celebration. Guests included only friends of John's parents and friends of his brother, John's birthday serving as ample reason for a party. With the arrival of the guests, John disappeared. My subsequent search for him ended when I found John in his bedroom intent on a game of solitaire. Asked why he didn't join the party, he shrugged, offering that everyone was just sitting around talking and drinking, that nothing much was going on anyway. Despite the fact that John, known as "the life of the party" in other circles (e.g., the social club of which he was a former member), is a great lover of social functions, his self-image precluded his seeing himself as fitting in with the group that was interacting in the living room in honor of his birthday. He thus excluded himself from an important arena of social learning, denying himself the experience of interacting with adult social groupings. In part, I would argue, the occasional "inappropriate" remarks or actions of which he is guilty when he does find himself in such groups can be traced back to the simple fact that he lacks experience within them.

This general constellation of elements that keeps John from including himself in adult activities similarly leads others to *exclude him* from activities in which he might otherwise participate. A straightforward example of this can be found in an incident that occurred while Lee and John were on vacation visiting family on the East coast. Dan, after taking care of some business in a neighboring city, joined them a few days after they arrived and immediately became acquainted with the three attractive young ladies down the street. After a sidewalk rendezvous, he extended an invitation to all three of them to join him for a night on the town, an invitation they promptly accepted. When John, aghast at the fact that Dan hadn't even thought of sharing his good fortune, confronted Dan the next morning with a demand for an explanation as to why he hadn't been included, Dan offered that he and his companions had spent most of the evening in bars and discotheques. Since John didn't drink, Dan explained that he had assumed John wouldn't be interested. John, a consummate dancer, could only comment to me a week later that if given the opportunity to join such a party, he would have learned how to drink and how to enjoy it on the spot.

While John's abstinence offered Dan a logical rationale for excluding him, his motivations for not including John in his foursome were certainly more complex. John, he knew, simply didn't have the social skills, to impress his three very impressionable new companions; drinking was only the most visible and obvious manifestation of this.

Dan, like his parents, is confused over the extent to which John's incompetence is physiologically based and the extent to which it is socially conditioned. In explaining John's shocking naiveté regarding the social and human context surrounding sexuality, for example, he provided a succinct definition of John's incompetence as being aggravated by limited experience with and exposure to ordinary social interaction. As such, his comment highlights the unique role played by the socialization process undergone by many mildly retarded individuals:

John's naiveté comes from the fact that he hasn't had enough social contact in the same way that you or I would in high school. He hasn't grown up with a peer group that's stable, you know? I mean, at a certain age everybody starts passing the word that chicks are neat to fuck or that they got tits or "Hey, this is happening!" And the guys who are interested are going, "Yeah!" and the guys who aren't interested are going, "I think there is something out there that I should be knowing about and I don't know why I don't". And about a month later it hits them and everybody's going, "Yeah!. Will you go out with me?" and the guys start chasing women. But John hasn't grown up with, with ... the same kind of chain of events. They haven't fallen into place at the proper times. That's what it looks like to me. So he's feeling the moves but he doesn't know what to do about it.

CONCLUSIONS

Admittedly, one example can in no way do justice to the complexity of John's experience. Isolating this one episode from its context has downplayed the way it interrelates with the countless other events which have made up his life — though attempts have been made to suggest the significance of such interrelationships. Further, the incidents mentioned tend to cloak the Hamlins in an aura of insensitive, cold malevolence. In truth, they are caring, concerned people who, in many ways, have enabled John to more nearly fulfill his potential, who do unquestionably want the best for him, and who believe that their actions are designed to fulfill that wish.

Even so, the analysis of this incident convincingly illustrates the pervasive effects of attitudes, adjusted expectations, and the consequent reorganized social milieu of a labeled individual as they impinge on that individual's competence. It has exposed the differential assumptions coloring the upbringing of a labeled individual and his unlabeled brother and has documented how these assumptions can and are translated into consequences. It has suggested that an individual's inability to develop normatively in certain spheres eventually leads to more generalized incompetence as he is denied the opportunity to learn behaviors that might be within the realm of his capabilities. As such, it has highlighted the necessity for increased attention to the socialization process undergone by mentally retarded individuals.

Further, analysis of this incident has emphasized the need for intensive research within small settings like the family if a complete understanding of the role played by socialization in shaping the lives of mentally retarded persons is to be gained. Large scale studies employing survey and questionnaire techniques tend to gloss the complexity of the interactions we have suggested here (should they uncover them at all); to fail to recognize the dichotomy between stated ideals of parents and others and their real actions; to ignore those details that elucidate attitudes, actions and their consequences and place them within a holistic context.

While not rejecting explanations which focus on retarded mental processes as providing the foundation for incompetence in their entirety, then, this paper suggests that the general competence of mildly retarded individuals is in part a function of the socialization process they have undergone. The focus in this particular critical incident has been the family. Parents, however, are not the only socialization agents an individual will confront. Mentally retarded people, in particular, seem to be exposed to a large number of significant others who also affect their continuing socialization experiences. Teachers, social workers, counselors, residential home caretakers are but a few of these. These care-givers constantly find themselves in the position of having to make decisions concerning what is right for their charges. Their decisions often overtly structure the opportunities of mildly retarded individuals to achieve a more normative level of competence. We cannot, at this point, control whatever biological factors might contribute to the incompetence of mildly retarded people. We can, however, control our own involvement in exacerbating that incompetence by having it spill over into areas where it need not exist. Admittedly, doing so is often difficult. Even individuals sensitive to respecting retarded individuals as adults find themselves slipping into behavior patterns that fall short of their ideal. Still, a greater appreciation of what mentally retarded individuals can learn and an equal appreciation of how socialization experiences provide or deny opportunities to learn will better enable the mildly retarded to adapt successfully in their communities.

ACKNOWLEDGEMENT

The preparation of this paper was made possible by the Mental Retardation Research Center, University of California at Los Angeles (USPHS Grant HD-04612-05), the Community Context of Normalization Study (NICHD Grant HD-09474-02), and by the Community Adaptation of Mildly Retarded Persons Study(USPHS 5 PO1 HD11944).

NOTES

1. Pseudonyms have been used, and identifying characteristics changed, in order to insure the anonymity of "John" and his family.
2. While data collection for the "Normalization" project formally ended in 1978, I have continued to maintain regular contact with John and his family through the present time.

REFERENCES

Becker, H. S.
  1963 *Outsiders. Studies in the sociology of deviance.* New York: The Free Press.
Blumer, H.
  1969 *Symbolic interactionism.* Englewood Cliffs, NJ: Prentice-Hall, Inc.
Cameron, M. O.
  1973 Identity and the shoplifter. *In* E. Rubington and M. S. Weinberg (eds.), *Deviance. The interactionist perspective.* New York: The Macmillan Co.
Damon, W. and Hart, D.
  1982 The development of self-understanding from infancy through adolescence. *Child Development, 53*: 841—864.
Edgerton, R. B.
  1975 Issues relating to the quality of life among mentally retarded persons. *In* M. J. Begab and S. A. Richardson (eds.), *The mentally retarded and society: A social science perspective.* Baltimore: University Park Press.
Edgerton, R. B. and Langness, L. L.
  1978 Observing mentally retarded persons in community settings: An anthropological perspective. *In* B. P. Sackett (ed.), *Observing Behavior, Volume I: Theory and application in mental retardation.* Baltimore: University Park Press.
Farber, B.
  1968 *Mental retardation: Its social context and social consequences.* Boston: Houghton Mifflin Co.
Filstead, W. J. (ed.).
  1972 *An introduction to deviance.* Chicago: Rand McNally College Publishing Company.

Goffman, E.
    1959 The moral career of the mental patient. *Psychiatry: Journal for the Study of Interpersonal Processes, 22*: 123—131.
Koegel, P.
    1981 Life history: A vehicle toward the holistic understanding of deviance. *Journal of Community Psychology, 9*: 162—176.
Langness, L. L. and Frank, G.
    1981 *Lives. An anthropological approach to biography.* Novato, CA: Chandler and Sharp.
Levine, H. G. and Langness, L. L.
    1983 Context ability and performance: Comparison of competitive athletics among mildly mentally retarded and nonretarded adults. *American Journal of Mental Deficiency, 87*(5): 528—538.
MacAndrew, C. and Edgerton, R. B.
    1969 *Drunken comportment: A social explanation.* Chicago: Aldine Publishing Co. London: T. Nelson and Sons.
Mead, G. H.
    1940 *Mind, self and society.* Chicago: University of Chicago Press.
Ray, M. B.
    1964 The cycle of abstinence and relapse among heroin addicts. *In* H. S. Becker (ed.), *The other side.* New York: The Free Press.
Reiss, A. J., Jr.
    1964 The social integration of queers and peers. *In* H. S. Becker (ed.), *The other side.* New York: The Free Press.
Rubington, E. and Weinberg, M. S. (eds.).
    1973 *Deviance. The interactionist perspective.* New York: The MacMillian Co.
Scheff, T. L.
    1966 *Being mentally ill: A sociological theory.* Chicago: Aldine Publishing Co.
Scott, R. A.
    1969 *The making of blind men.* New York: Russell Sage Foundation.
Turner, J. L.
    1980 Yes I am human: Autobiography of a "retarded career". *Journal of Community Psychology, 8*: 3—8.

IT WASN'T FAIR: SIX YEARS IN THE LIFE OF LARRY B.

> I took her out/It wasn't fair fair fair
> Sat by another man in my place/It wasn't fair fair fair
> Took her out/It wasn't fair fair fair
> Bought her a hamburger/It wasn't fair
> It wasn't fair, it wasn't fair, it wasn't fair
> Sat by another man in my place.
>
> *Lyric by Larry B.*

The above is only one of the many songs composed by Larry B. who aspires to become a rock star. Born November 3, 1950, Larry was the first child of the B's; his father was a mechanic and his mother a laboratory technician at the time, a job she had to abandon to care to Larry. Hyperactive as a toddler, Larry was taken by his mother to a child guidance clinic at the University of Southern California when he was three years of age. He was then diagnosed as having "possible minimal brain damage". He was examined by a number of psychiatrists and psychologists and did not appear to them as retarded although they agreed that he was definitely hyperactive. At approximately $4\frac{1}{2}$ years Larry became verbal and was placed in a special school which attempted to train autistic and emotionally disturbed children. When Larry was 7 he was placed in an elementary school class for the educable mentally retarded although the school psychologist "didn't know if he belonged there". His hyperactivity caused considerable disruption at school and finally he was allowed to remain through the lunch hour only when his mother agreed to come and supervise him. He somehow made it through the grades, learning to read when he was 8 or 9. When he finished the elementary program he was sent to a Junior High School which did not have an EMR Program but did have "lower index" classes. Although here certain teachers took time to work with him, he was sufficiently atypical to suffer relentless teasing from his schoolmates, a state of affairs which seems to have remained constant through High School as well. There, in his final year of school, he suffered a complete nervous breakdown, for which he was institutionalized. He was awarded a certificate rather than a diploma.

It is clear from all sources that Larry's adolescence was his most tumultuous period. Not only a constant target of ridicule and rejection at school, he also became acutely aware of how different he was being treated when compared with his younger sister. In fact, his institutionalization followed a series of violent incidents against his parents' property, which Larry performed because he felt they treated his younger sister as more adult than he and, as he disclosed to us, he wanted to "fair" them. After twice being

65

L. L. Langness and H. G. Levine (eds.), Culture and Retardation, 65—80.

committed to mental health institutions for periods of one to two months, Larry moved out of his parent's home and into a board and care facility. After one apparently very unpleasant year there he moved into Hillhouse, the board and care facility where he lived when he was first contacted in July of 1976 by our researchers. He was followed by Laura, an attractive fieldworker of approximately his own age until September of 1978. He was recontacted in August of 1980 and followed by Ted, again almost his same age, until February of 1982. We have maintained only minimal contact with him since that time. During this approximately six year period Larry completed an independence training program and moved from the board and care facility into his own apartment. This apparent success story is worth examining as is the record of Larry's life during this time, a life that can be described as centering around 5 rather obsessive and related concerns: stardom, sex, companionship, loneliness, and retardation.

First, it must be acknowledged that it is quite likely that Larry is not really retarded at all. He does demonstrate in all interactions a basic linguistic competence; he has the ability to read, add, subtract, judge time, make calculations, and can, in general, "take care of himself". He has no visible handicap and is, in fact, a fairly attractive blond, blue-eyed young man. Nonetheless, he has been picked up by the California delivery system and classified as retarded and thus, like many other such cases, must be considered in any discussion of the mildly retarded population.

It is clear that Larry has some type of mental problem. He is subject to episodes in which he becomes highly agitated, his language becomes disjointed, and his associations can become quite bizarre. Indeed, his presence at all times is bizarre in that he speaks in an inappropriately loud and monotonous nasal voice and is conversationally aggressive, often broaching quite personal subjects in most inappropriate situations. Although he attempts to rationalize his behavior his reasoning is often blatantly false.

STARDOM

Larry attributes his past mental breakdown to "trying too hard to be famous". He is obsessed with the idea of becoming a famous rock star and periodically sends tapes of his music to people in the music business. Unfortunately, he has so little ability, he never receives a reply of any kind other than a polite acknowledgement. Larry is fascinated by the "business end" of stardom and fantasizes what it would be like to be a big star. He would live in a big house, he would have no privacy, he would have people to cook for him, manage his money, etc. An example of the flavor of this can be seen in the following statement to Laura while he was still in the board and care home:

In here they have people who cook for you. This is a place for famous people. All famous people live here and the people in the office help the famous people manage their money. The cook is to cook for the famous people who live here. So the people you see here are famous.

To Laura's sarcastic "Come on, Larry", Larry responded immediately with "face up to reality", acknowledging the fantasy. But it is not entirely fantasy for Larry. It is obvious that he both reflects on it and attempts to bring it about. This can be seen in his demonstration tapes, in his continual attempt at song writing, in his periodic attempts to either explain that some people like his music and others don't, or why "it is no fun to be famous". For example, in a conversation with Ted, Larry explains that a star's tax bracket is so high they only have "$25,000 a year to live on". And, with a star's expenses, "$25,000 doesn't go very far". He continues with, "There's no point in being famous because you're just going to fade after a while". He works hard to convince himself that performing for money isn't the only important thing. "I'm just as happy performing for friends as Elton John is performing concerts. I'm just as happy doing a speech on that tape with you (Ted) as the Beatles are doing a speech on the radio to T.V. I'm just as happy making my money off custodial work as the Rolling Stones are making money off their music." When Ted questions Larry as to how he knows this: "Well, I work and get paid, right? The Rolling Stones make money off their music and that's a job to them." Larry adds, "When I don't work I feel 'yichy' ". But he never really gives up hope. After this remark he sings the following song:

> As I look out my window, I see red leaves
> And the birds are singing
> And I see a white tree-trunk
> And the cat chased the Blue Jay up the tree
> To protect my mother's hummingbird feeder
> And the red leaves blow in the wind
> And the birds are singing
> And I see a white tree trunk

Larry asks Ted "did you hear how long I held that last note?" Ted acknowledges that he did and Larry queries, "It doesn't sound good enough for a club does it?" When Ted asks Larry why he never sings any new tunes Larry assures him that "he works hard at his craft every day", and he composes so many songs he "seldom has time to memorize them". Ted asks to see a new song (Larry has the words and chords which are noted on a sheet of ruled notebook paper):

> I'm free like always
> I travel the road
> How neat, too
> I did a dance north of where I live on stage
> I was forced to do so
> I sing a song in Burbank, two songs

Ted asks Larry to explain it: "I'm free because I'm unknown and so I won't be mobbed. Sometimes I do dances for friends when they invite me to. I sang some songs for friends." Ted asks how his friends like his songs and is confronted with the following: "Some of them liked it and some of them liked it fairly well and some of them like it. And some of them just liked it fairly well." Larry then adds: "A few people thought it was out of date. They're into punk rock now. You heard of punk rock? It's mainly older people who like my music." Later in this same conversation Larry explains: "See, for instance, I sound good to friends, but not to the public. When I sing for friends, I sound fairly good, but if I sing for the public, I sound way off key." "Why is that?" Ted asks. "Because my talent is not employable talent", Larry replies and then continues: "As well as with the guitar. See, my guitar sounds o.k. to friends, but to the public it would sound off key." "Would friends put up with more than the public?" "In a way", Larry responds, "I might be a string or two off for friends, but I would sound four strings off to the public". "Why is that so?" "Because I wasn't born with professional talent . . . because I took up singing too late."

Larry first took up the guitar in High School and got the idea of composing from the Beatles. He was also attracted to the music of the Monkees about whom he says, "They faded and now they're unknown like you and me and probably have to work now". When Ted asks what Larry writes most of his songs about he is told: "Love and nature. How I feel being unknown; how I feel being where I'm at." Interestingly, although Ted asserts elsewhere in his notes that Larry has a "tin ear", is an "awful guitarist", "a pretty poor singer", and that his guitar work is "eccentric at best", he also allows that "it's during periods like this that I like Larry a whole lot". Ted also feels that Larry's songs reveal much more about him that any number of interviews. "Larry, the songwriter", Ted says, "talks a lot about the pain he's suffered in relationships, particularly, it appears, in his relationships with women. This is simply illustrated, I think, in the following song entitled *She Don't Wanna Dance With Me*:"

> Went to the club/Met a beautiful chick
> Said, "You wanna dance with me?"
> She said, "Sorry, I have a bad hip".
> Which is a lie . . .
> She don't wanna dance with me.

Larry's songs tend to be literal and based upon actual experiences. He is often rejected. In still another song the most telling line is "She don't like me a bit", which leads to another of the major themes in his life, his constant desire to find a girlfriend which, although it does have an important sexual component, is of much more significance than merely a desire for sex.

SEX

As an example of Larry's aggressive and inappropriate conversational style, as well as of his interest in sex and finding a girlfriend, We quote the following from Laura's very first interview with him:

Larry: Do you have sex with men?
Laura: Yes. Do you have sex with women?
Larry: Yes. Do they use a rubber?
Laura: No. Do you use a rubber?
Larry: No. I take it out before. Do you take the pill after having sex?
Laura: Yes. I am married.
Larry: Oh. Do you kiss other men?
Laura: My husband would take a dim view of that. Do you still want to be in this study?
Larry: Yes.

This first encounter is described by Laura as Larry challenging her and *vice versa*. Larry continues this approach, at times even more inappropriately, throughout the more than two years Laura worked with him. Two months later, after Laura has seen him several times, Larry opens the door to his apartment for her dressed only in his undershorts. She waits outside and during the course of the later interview the following exchange occurs:

Larry: Is it wrong to kiss another guy?
Laura: It isn't important what I think about it, it's more important if you think it is o.k.
Larry: Did you ever kiss another girl?
Laura: Yes.
Larry: Have you ever finger-banged another woman?
Laura: I don't think that's any of your business!
Larry: That's because it's private, huh?

As part of her fieldwork with Larry, Laura asked him to keep a diary for her. Among the early entries he gave her:

September 2, 1976:
   I went to Par workshop. Kiss a girl on a job and got scolded. Without anyone knowing, I felt her out during breaks (sic). They only found out I kissed her.
September 4, 1976:
   I visited my mother, I called my girlfriend (Suzi) and we really love each other, I've gotten to be happy with her. Our love has developed. (On questioning it is revealed that "Suzi is everyone's girlfriend because she's not ready to go with one guy. She's nice and friendly.")
September 5, 1976:
   I went to visit the Wildwood Gardens, jacked off with a friend, kissed him on the lips.

Although the diary entries change after this, Larry follows a short time later by volunteering his experiences with a prostitute he met at the beach. Then later he leads Laura into a discussion of his (male) roommates' nice legs, and "hot pants", and follows this with questions about gay bars, picking up gay, and his homosexual experiences in general. Larry confesses that with men, "It turns my stomach to kiss them. I would rather do that with girls. I find it more relaxing. Wouldn't it turn your stomach to do it with another woman?" He then describes for her in intimate detail a recent homosexual encounter from which he extricated himself by claiming (falsely) to have hemorrhoids. Larry's baiting of Laura comes to an end towards the last of her fieldwork with a rather hilarious phone call in which he demands to know if she thinks Hollywood prostitutes will take a check. Laura answers that they will not, nor will they take credit cards. Larry concludes with, "They won't accept money orders, that's for damn sure".

There is little doubt that Larry was challenging Laura to set limits and that his aggressive sexual talk was deliberately provocative. This is clear when one understands that this type of behavior does not constitute part of Larry's repertoire during the 18 months he was followed by Ted. When he does discuss sex with Ted it is a serious discussion, "man to man", in which Larry confesses to his 3 real heterosexual encounters, once with a prostitute and twice with a girl he had known previously. Larry indicates that sex with a prostitute was unrewarding because he had to pay and there was no relationship established. He asks Ted about his relationship, sexual and otherwise, with his wife. In the context of the discussion this was not considered by Ted to be inappropriate.

It should not be inferred from the above that Larry's interest in Laura was only or even primarily sexual. The sexual maneuvering is in fact only one part of a broader attempt to set limits with Laura and to determine her availability as a girlfriend. As this is intimately tied to Larry's concern with his retardation and self-image and how this relates to his loneliness, it needs to be seen in that context.

COMPANIONSHIP

Larry's very first question of Laura, which eventually led to the question about her sex life, was "Do you think I am immature?" Laura replies that she doesn't know him well enough to make such a judgment. His next question is "Do you think I am good looking?" Laura says "yes" and Larry asks her what that means. She replies that it means "attractive". His next question is "What does emotionally handicapped mean?" These are all questions that Larry comes back to time after time either in this form or in similar ways.

In the next interview Larry comes right to the point:

". . . If you wasn't married, would you be too mature for me to marry?"
"I think so because I am older than you" (she is four years older).
"How about if you were the same age, would you still be too mature?"
"I don't know, I am not so . . ."
"So I don't have to worry about it, right?"
"Right, What makes you ask a question like that?"
"I am looking for a girlfriend."

"Don't you think it would be nice to find out whether or not you liked the person before you consider marrying them?"

"Yeah. But how do you find a girlfriend?"

Laura explains that she went out with men, dated, and flirted. Larry asks, "Sexually?" He then tells her that he once had a girlfriend for 11 months but they broke up "because we didn't have enough in common". He then asks her again what it means to say someone is emotionally handicapped. From there he goes on to discuss her "maturity" and the fact that he "hasn't had the experiences most guys my age have". His lack of maturity and sophistication is a continuing theme. He talks to the waitresses where he eats but never asks them out as he says he is "too shy" and "they are too sophisticated for me in the first place because I am not exactly mature for my age and I have learning disabilities". In fact, Larry often picks his restaurants because the waitresses are friendly and will talk to him.

There is virtually no extended interview or conversation with either Laura or Ted over the entire 6 year period that does not deal in one way or another with the handicap/girlfriend/loneliness themes that almost always go together. He dwells on his past girlfriend, reporting that "If your girlfriend breaks up with you, there is nothing you can do". This also repeatedly takes the form of "you can't force a girl to love you if she doesn't".

In one of the early interviews with Laura, Larry suddenly announces for no apparent reason: "I am not retarded! I think everyone has learning disabilities in one area or another, do you agree?" Laura agrees and Larry admits that he, too, has learning disabilities. Later in the same day when Laura asks him a question he demands to know: "You don't think I am retarded do you?" He then discusses the retarded people he has known and points out that they "can't tell the difference between personal and non-personal questions" and they act "childishly". In a subsequent interview he reminds Laura that she told him her project was for slightly retarded people and wants to know if that is true. When she replies that it is, he defines retardation for her: "Learning disabilities, brain damage or brain defect". Laura asks him if being retarded bothered him. Larry replies, "No, I am used to my handicap. I have learned to enjoy it and be happy with it." When asked which of the 3 categories he belongs in he replies "learning disabilities". When asked specifically what that means to him, personally: "It means that no one will hire me on a job unless they hear from a Rehab counselor or social worker. Get what I mean when I say it is hard for handicapped people to find a job?" Larry had previously complained that night clubs didn't hire retarded people and that was one reason he couldn't be a "star".

Even after months of the researcher/client relationship Larry is still testing.

"Yeah", Larry says, "if you went with a retarded person you couldn't relate to him could you?"

"What do you mean, 'went with'?"

"If you went steady with a retarded person, you couldn't relate to him very well could you? You would be under a lot of strain. Like if you went with me, you would be under a lot of strain and you would get ulcers. You'd be under pressures and that wouldn't be very pleasant."

"I don't understand why you would say that. In any case our relationship is one of researcher and . . ."

"Just good friends", Larry replies, "and you are too sophisticated for me".

Larry's life is a constant quest for a girlfriend and companionship but he is often inhibited because of his "lack of sophistication". About a new, attractive addition to the board and care home he reports he did not consider her a prospective date because "She's been out in the world more than me". He broods over his lost girlfriend and has violent fantasies about her. Here is an excerpt from Laura's field notes:

With a gush of words, Larry describes his fantasies of harming his ex-girlfriend, Sally S. (He also phoned her on several occasions to discuss these very same fantasies.) Once in a while, he declared, he gets these fantasies of harming Sally but as soon as he remembers that he would go to jail for it, he claims he gets over it. (I don't believe that statement and I don't think he really does either.) His fantasies of harming Sally stem from the fact that she hurt him when she left him. he hopes he will only have these 'flashbacks' (of harming her) until he finds another girlfriend. He is not going to act out his fantasies because he would be put in jail and "being there for one night is just as bad as being there for 20 years". His fantasies are: "hitting her or burning her face or stabbing her mother for calling the police for hitting her. But if I do any of that, I would surely go to jail and never get out. (Smiled). And if I do anything that is half-death or full death, that is the same thing. But if I do something that is just wound but not murder it would be at least 10 years. Let's put it this way, being in jail for a day is just as bad as being there for 30 years."

It occurred to me that Larry might be lonely and that might account for why he had been thinking a lot about Sally S. lately. He indulged my question and considered the fact that he does have people to talk with, while realizing that doesn't stop him from being lonely. Larry admitted, "he's lonely for a girl". Abruptly he changed the subject and told me he wanted to talk about good things now. Good things include the fact that "all men find girls who are too sophisticated for them and all women find men who are too sophisticated for them". Again he confirmed in his own mind, with my help, that a relationship with me (a woman too sophisticated for him) is not an option. "Sophisticated means that you cannot relate to them. That means you don't have enough in common with them."

Later in their relationship Larry asks Laura if he could employ the Mafia to "beat up my ex-girlfriend". Still later he mentions the possibility of throwing acid in her face (he apparently had seen this on television) and also discusses the possibility of rape if you can't get a girl to like you. Three and a half years later Larry still reports the same type of violent fantasies, again triggered by a conversation about Sally S. Three years after they broke up Larry called her and she hung up. He then phoned the police. When Ted asks him why he called the police he replies, "Because she left me and I couldn't find another girlfriend . . . I wanted her back." Larry apparently thought the police could order her to stay with him: "They could say, you keep going from one man onto another. Just say with one and keep goin' and quit goin' with so many different men." Larry returns to this theme of being rejected over and over again in conversations with both Laura and Ted. Sometimes he discusses hitting her over the head with a bottle, sometimes cutting her face with a broken bottle, sometimes acid in the face, always reasoning that ". . . other men wouldn't find her attractive so she'd have to come back to me". After recounting some of these violent fantasies Larry sometimes adds, "Now you know what it feels like to be retarded". Ted asks Larry what an ideal marriage would be like: "Oh, sleeping in the same bed together. Enjoying one another. Cooking for your wife. Having her cook for you. Helping her clean the house. Helping her do the laundry instead of having her do all the shit by herself. Helping her keep house, helping her shop for food. Cooking for her when she's sick. Taking care of her and spending the whole day with her when she's sick. 'Cause you can't do your hobby when you're taking care of your wife. Her illness is more important than my guitar. You know what I mean, don't you?"

Larry, of course, has never had such a relationship and is in fact chronically and excruciatingly lonely.

LONELINESS

Loneliness is a theme that constantly recurs in both Laura's and Ted's fieldnotes about Larry. Some idea of the depths of Larry's feelings about this can be seen in the fact that he tends to pick restaurants on the basis of whether or not the waitresses are friendly and talk to him rather than for other more usual reasons. Similarly, in his attempts to keep a diary for Laura the entries are always very brief and recount over and over little more than how he got up, went for coffee, took a shower or nap, played his guitar, period. He regards napping as an antidote for boredom and often naps one or two hours per day. He has few friends and sees them only sporadically. He wishes for a roomate at times but concludes that good roommates are hard to find, and he really would prefer a girlfriend. He pines for a former girlfriend and asks Ted if he can read him a "story". It goes as follows:

> My first girlfriend died.
> She drowned.
> That made me mad and sad.
> We planned to get married as soon as we turned 18, we're the same age.
> She died three years before we were old enough to get married.

This story is entitled "Girlfriend". According to Larry's mother there really was such a girl (when Larry was about 15 years old) who drowned and Larry had gone with her for some time and was terribly upset by it. When Ted asks him why he had written the story Larry replies, "just memories", then adds, "Do you think I'll ever find another girlfriend?"

In only her second interview with Larry, Laura is asked, "Do you know how I handle my loneliness?" He tells her "Well, I find things I like to do and, like for instance on weekends, you know if I am not doing anything on weekends, you know, I go for a walk". He continues, "I stop in a restaurant and I have coffee. I come home and do things I like to do. I nap."

On other occasions Larry reports that as a cure for loneliness, he talks to friends, he walks, he naps, he plays his guitar, he gets coffee, he watches the leaves fall, and, finally on one occasion, he reports that he went outside "to count the leaves!" He reflects on his past girlfriends and broods over finding a new one. His loneliness is linked in his mind to his "handicap", but it is exacerbated by his move from a board and care home to his own apartment which is the context in which we see the interplay of these four themes with his fifth obsessional concern, his retardation.

RETARDATION

In 1976, when Laura first begins her work with Larry, he is living in a board and care facility with a roomate and is involved in "Independence training for young adults". The goal of this training for Larry and for the teachers is to get him living independently in the community in his own apartment. He tells her the first day she meets him that "I would like to get an apartment but I can't because I don't have the money or a job". He gets $309 per month from SSI and believes he can get some kind of training. He takes cooking lessons and is waiting for a job in a sheltered workshop doing piece work. Although the cooking lessons are to teach him to cook for himself Larry fantasizes that he might someday be able to get a job as a cook.

Larry's concern with his handicap is clear from the first day when he begins by asking Laura if she thinks he is immature, then if she thinks he is emotionally handicapped. In their next meeting he asks her what "rehabilitation center" means and he returns to his immaturity and emotional handicap. He also tells her about the "living in apartment group" he attended and what he learned (paying rent, contact gas company, etc.), and also about learning how to market for himself. He tells her, "I am tired of living in board and care homes. They are for sick people. They are depressing. I want to live independently." He returns to the theme of his immaturity and then for the first time mentions that he has "learning disabilities". Then at the end of this interview Larry asks her what mentally retarded means and answers his own question with "it means a person has brain damage". He asks Laura if *she* thinks he is mentally retarded and she replies that he told her himself that he has learning disabilities.

On the very next interview the first topic of conversation is Larry's mental health. He says that because he isn't depressed anymore he took a shower "for the first time in a long time". (Larry had been on a drug that made him depressed and his prescription had just been changed). He quit his job at the workshop because he didn't think it was fair to pay on a piece work basis.

Now he takes a class entitled "Job Readiness". During this period he constantly refers to the board and care home as a "nut house" and his room as a "cell". At this point he also meets a new counselor who is black and who tells him that "everyone has a handicap", and one just has to overcome the handicap. This counselor's handicap is that he is black, a claim Larry regards with suspicion. But he begins to question Laura on this point. "Does everyone have a handicap?" etc. He lands a job as a part-time janitor in a school and starts a checking account.

A month later Larry announces to Laura that he is not retarded and that "everyone has learning disabilities in one area or another . . ." He then tells her that he believes he became mentally ill when he was about 11 and then again when he was about 15. He announces that he has not been attending his "Group" because "it is just a mental health facility for young adults that have mental problems". He apparently felt there were "too many people yelling at each other and I just couldn't take all that violence". He returns to his claim of not being retarded and argues that the board and care home is now a hospital. Larry also wants to know if "sisters could really put spells on people" because when he was sick at age 14 his sister threatened to put a spell on him. He claims to have started believing in "genies and other imaginary people".

In November of 1976 Larry is hospitalized for a few days as a result of a screaming and yelling fit in the board and care home. He was self-admitted and apparently had complained of dizziness and stiffness. It was believed this was a reaction to the Haldol he had been taking. Two weeks later he is concerned over his behavior in becoming obsessed with asking a question and then repeating it over and over again and then getting all "worked up". He describes how irritated the staff at the board and care facility become when he does this. But he has now signed the papers for Project AHEAD (a pseudonym for an independent living program) and although he is highly agitated he is excited about the move to an apartment. He literally yells at Laura: "I need a change to live in an apartment! You can understand that, can't you!" At the same time that he expresses complete happiness about the move he also reports that he is very tense and worries a lot. A psychologist has told him that "he worries too much about the past and the future that he can't enjoy the present", a phrase he repeats over and over again (repeating things is one of the characteristics that causes people to describe Larry as boring).

In January of 1977, still at the board and care home, Larry reports that the purpose of his job readiness program is "to get a job so I can work myself out of the cuckoo's nest". His leaving is being held up while they try to locate a roomate for him. He is "worried about it". He believes his apartment might be "real cozy, rugged, beautiful and colorful" but he hasn't seen it yet. He reports that "it is in a real nice neighborhood". He returns to the theme of retardation and demands to know if Laura's project deals with "slightly retarded people". When she acknowledges that it does he defines it as previously mentioned and claims to be "used to his handicap". Again he discusses how Laura would be under stress if she went with a retarded person.

In the next interview which takes place in a restaurant Larry conspicuously lowers his voice every time he mentions the word retarded. He wants to know why it is that every time he sees Laura he asks her if her project deals with the retarded. He is concerned that people can tell he is retarded by looking at him. A short time later he comes up with a new self-definition: "do you remember I told you I wasn't exactly mature for my age? I think I was being hard on myself when I said I was emotionally immature because I think everyone is emotional to a certain degree. I think everyone has some craziness in them. I think everyone is immature up to a certain degree and I even think everyone has some child(ish)ness in them. I even think everyone has a certain amount of retardation in them. I even think that people have a little hoodishness in them. They get a little smart alecky or sneaky or slightly delinquent at times." Larry claims to have heard this from a psychologist in the past and says he is "finally ready to admit it instead of being hard on myself".

Larry returns to the theme of retardation over and over, comparing himself to others and variously claiming that he either can or cannot relate to the retarded, that someone who is not retarded can not date someone who is, that "everyone has a handicap", that he "doesn't mind working with the retarded" but they are "not geared to his level", and so on. Eventually he fastens on the label "developmentally disabled" which he defines as a person who "lacks the right brain chemistry". Now he is taking a "social skills" class where he learns to "shake hands with people and not stare at them". He tells Laura now that the whole idea of board and care is to prepare one to live in the outside world and asks her if she thinks he could live in his own apartment. According to Larry, if one holds down a full time job and makes good money there is no point in living in a board and care facility. When he gets a full time job he plans not to live off SSI anymore as people on SSI receive it because they are mentally ill or have a physical illness. Now he does not see himself as truly handicapped. At least he's not handicapped like a person "who goes around with a red and white cane and is blind", or "in a wheelchair or holding on to stilts when they walk, or carrying their legs with them when they walk on their arms". He concludes with, "I just see myself as a regular individual with just a minor handicap like just about any other person in the world. Like you and me. I don't see myself as handicapped or emotional. I just see myself as a regular person."

At the end of March there still is no apartment available for Larry. Larry now announces that the board and care facility is "not a coo-koo's nest" and that he shouldn't call it that. He asks her unexpectedly if he "still talks loud". She acknowledges that he does but adds that it only bothers her in restaurants. He also wants to know if his mother seemed strict to her and then discusses his relationship with her which is basically positive. When Larry runs out of his pills (Artans) he does not get the prescription refilled and explains he won't have withdrawal symptoms "because he is used to holding down a job" (he is still janitoring in the school). Laura can't make the connection so Larry explains "Not experiencing withdrawal is due to being able to hold down an outside job, as you are in good mental health. If your mental health has improved then you are used to having it improved, you don't react to not taking medication." On a later occasion Larry tells Laura that after he graduates from Project AHEAD "he won't be mentally disabled because he will have a job on the outside".

Eventually, through Project AHEAD, Larry does get an apartment with a roomate. One month they get an award as "tenants of the month". When Laura asks him how he thinks he has changed he replies, "I used to compare myself to other people and I don't do that anymore. I used to compare myself and get angry." "Because you don't measure up?" "Yes, I don't measure up to guys my age because I've been in board and care."

At this point Larry is seeing a psychiatrist once a month and two social workers one of which is with project AHEAD. He thinks he can do without a doctor "because he has reached the point where he can help himself". He offers a classification of his residences for Laura in chronological order:

1. Safenook — a hospital
2. Eastside Arms — a low class nest
3. Resthaven — a high class nest
4. Northside — a hospital (it is the hospital he was in briefly when he apparently mixed marijuana with his other drugs)
5. Westgate — a high class cuckoo's nest. "It's between a hospital and an apartment."
6. Project AHEAD — "A training apartment because you do your own cooking, shopping, paying the bills, etc."

Larry reports that he has "forgiven his Mom for taking him to a 'funny farm' because she took him out and to Project AHEAD".

In fact, Larry is doing very well in Project AHEAD. He is ranked second from the top of his class. He is reported to have done something no other student had ever done — he called the Project Supervisor and told him he had an *idea*. His idea was that workshops were poorly run and did nothing for the clients they were supposed to serve. The supervisor was impressed and mentioned Larry's remark to the vocational class the following day. This led to a discussion of having the tenants publish their own newsletter (nothing came of this).

In January of 1978, it is felt that Larry is about ready to leave Project AHEAD and progress to a job where he could earn $4.57 per hour on the maintenance crew of a large company. Larry is doing much better with his star fixation ever since one of the Project social workers had him bring his guitar and play for the other clients. They told him he was terrible and couldn't possibly make a living at it. Larry has been on time consistently and is believed to be highly motivated to successfully complete the program. He will have to find another apartment when he finishes as the Project AHEAD apartments have to be made available for new clients.

By August Larry reports that he still has to graduate from three classes: budgeting, cooking and leisure time. He is still doing well. He tells Laura that in 1974–75 he was "floating in a child's world" and now he is living in an adult world. He claims he got sick because he tried too hard to become famous. Although he is still thinking of his ex-girlfriend and wanting to "throw gasoline in her face" he is otherwise doing very well.

In December of 1979, Larry called Laura to report that he had moved into an apartment by himself and to give her his new address and phone number. In reference to the move Larry said, "I can handle myself. I have proved it."

Larry was living in this apartment in August of 1980 when Ted first contacted him. Their initial conversation consisted primarily of a monologue in which Larry told Ted how he has "come to grips with reality". He piles one platitude on another to the point where Ted writes in his notes, "It was much like reading all of Rod McKuen's books back to back".

Larry reports "The world's mean. The world's unfair. The world's a rip off. The future takes care as it comes. Life is a continuous change. It moves on. I've been through the whole pick. I've been through a lot of shit, but I've learned how to cope with it. You have to make a foundation before you build a wall and you have to build a roof," etc.

Larry is lonely and tells Ted in their first and virtually all subsequent interviews how much he wants to find a girlfriend. Loneliness is the primary theme during the approximately 16 months Ted worked with him but he also returned again and again to the familiar topics of stardom, companionship, and his retardation. The aggressive sexual conversations are absent in Larry's conversations with Ted. In his final interviews Larry reports that he is so lonely he wants to move back to the board and care facility!

From the point of view of those who were responsible for Larry's training and development Larry has to be seen as a success. He successfuly completed all of the various courses he needed; he learned how to shop, cook, work, and live independently, and, indeed, was often at the top of his class. Although he had his moments of anxiety he made the transition from board and care to supervised apartment to independent apartment just as was intended. From a different perspective, however, Larry's case must be seen as a failure as he now for the first time actually admits to and claims to accept his retardation and wants to give up his hard won independence to return to board and care. His excruciating loneliness defeats him in the end.

Underlying the particulars of Larry's life and the themes which characterize his personal history is a more general pattern we find in the mildly retarded. It begins with an ambiguous diagnosis. At times Larry is described as hyperactive; having minimal brain damage, an educably mentally retarded, emotionally disturbed and/or learning disabled. This is further compounded by the fact that he is a normal appearing fairly attractive young man. There is much marital conflict centering around his competency as he grows up. This ambiguity and conflict enables Larry to disavow his handicap, at least the most threatening label of mentally retarded, as he searches for an acceptable social identity and a meaningful way of accounting for his apparent differences from others. He rejects any peer affiliation with other retarded persons and his peers, in turn, dislike him because he thinks he is better than they are. He turns to the fantasy of being a rock star which, he believes, would help solve his problem. Everyone would adore him, he could hire people to care for him, and he would be a famous celebrity. As his lack of talent becomes increasingly difficult for him to deny, his self-aggrandizement becomes more difficult to sustain. At the same time he attempts to initiate and maintain social relationships with non-handicapped persons, to find a normal girlfriend and to get and maintain attention from the fieldworkers. As this cannot be entirely satisfactory he broods over his rejections and engages in violent fantasies of revenge which focus on the one apparently most traumatic rejection he experienced. He is forced to search for intimacy with anonymous and fleeting relationships with waitresses and homosexual encounters which he does not find satisfactory.

In spite of his apparent success in living independently it is clear that Larry cannot find the companionship and life that he so optimistically sought. His obsession with stardom, his loud and monotonous conversations, and his inappropriate behavior all combine to maintain his appearance of being retarded or otherwise mentally handicapped. Although the various courses he completed helped with the mechanics of living independently, they did not change his fundamentally inappropriate interactive strategies. His failure to find a girlfriend is a tragedy only partly of his own making. For most of the time Larry was observed a retarded girlfriend would not have been acceptable to him. But he most probably could not have found a "normal" girlfriend as his obsessions and demeanor so clearly stigmatized him. Even so, both Laura and Ted could empathize with him and they both report that he was at times "likeable". They do not feel it would have been impossible for him to find a companion of some kind. But this leads to further considerations. Where could he look? Living on his own Larry is not very mobile. He has only the bus for transportation. He has limited funds. He also has nowhere to go. He has already attended the various groups and activities provided for the handicapped and found them unrewarding. He has virtually no friends or acquaintances and rarely visits the one or two he does have. His mother, apparently to preserve her marriage, became increasingly distant (Larry's father never wanted anything to do with him) even as she encouraged Larry in his independence. Thus Larry is driven to choose his restaurants on the basis of whether or not the waitresses are friendly and will talk to him. As he doesn't understand the cultural rules about tipping and conversation and tries inappropriately to engage the waitresses in conversation, even they quickly reject him. In his desperation Larry goes out "to count the leaves" and to compose his songs of love and sadness ... "It wasn't fair, it wasn't fair". Indeed, it would seem that it wasn't. It would appear that what Larry really needed for "success" simply cannot be taught with our existing technology and knowledge as it requires an understanding of both cultural context and individual need which is, as yet, not available.

KEITH T. KERNAN, LINDA HUBBARD, AND KRISTINA KENNANN

LIVING IN THE REAL WORLD: PROCESS AND CHANGE
IN THE LIFE OF A RETARDED MAN

The adaptation of a mentally retarded person to a life in the community is an important issue that has been the focus of much scholarly research. Edgerton (1983) has reviewed the literature that attempts to assess such adaptation and reports that not only have multiple criteria been used for judging whether adaptation is successful or not, but also that there are disagreements about these findings. He concludes that "we know far too little about the processes of community adaptation to allow ourselves the illusion that we have already measured success or failure. It is far more likely that we will never know how to do so" (1983: 141).

A seemingly pessimistic conclusion, but if we interpret Edgerton correctly, he is saying that judgments of successful adaptations to life in the community are not likely to be informative or of much use if they are based on such simple, "objective" criteria as the avoidance of reinstitutionalization. Certainly there can be no pronouncements by fiat of what an acceptable quality of life would be for all individuals in all situations. Adjustment and adaptation to life in the community must not be considered as static states of achievement to be measured by tests, life satisfaction inventories, engagement in competitive employment, proper performance of daily duties as judged by social workers, and so on (Kernan and Koegel, 1984). Adjustment and adaptation, by their very nature, must be considered in terms of *process* and *change* (Edgerton, 1984: 2—3). Success or failure depends on the processes by which particular individuals adapt in distinctive ways to specific cultural milieus. Only by discovering how and why individuals develop particular styles of adaptation can we ever hope to judge whether or not they have been successful in their adaptation. Even more importantly, it is only through the understanding of these complex processes that we can ever hope to design programs that more effectively promote successful community life for the handicapped.

Studies are needed, then, that describe the lives of these people as they are lived on a daily basis, question how the individuals themselves feel about their lives, and examine how they go about achieving their various goals and desires. Many scholars have used life history methodology and analysis in elucidating questions about change, adaptation, conformity to societal expectations, and individual innovation (Crapanzano, 1980; Hughes, 1974; Kennann, 1984; Kennedy, 1977; Mandelbaum, 1973). These studies have demonstrated that the course of peoples' lives and the daily activities of those lives are determined by a number of factors: childhood experiences (Crapanzano, 1980; Frank, 1981; Hughes, 1974); the social and cultural mileu in

L. L. Langness and H. G. Levine (eds.), Culture and Retardation, 81—99.

which lives are being lived (Kennedy, 1977; Mandelbaum, 1973; Wilson, 1975); a sense of self worth and efficacy (Frank, 1981; Mintz, 1974; Wilson, 1975); crisis events (Erikson, 1975; Kaufman, 1981; Riegel, 1974); and short and long term goals, both realistic and unattainable (Kennan, 1984; Kennedy, 1977; Kuper, 1978). These and other aspects of the life process interact in complex ways, influencing the way people lead their lives and the changes that occur in their lives. The life course is a developmental process, and as such, it includes change (Buhler and Massarik, 1968; Dailey, 1971; Erikson, 1975). The changes that occur during a person's lifetime may be chosen by the person involved, or imposed by outside sources (Mandelbaum, 1973; Mintz, 1974); they may occur suddenly, or be long in developing (Crapanzano, 1980; Kennedy, 1977); they may be perceived as major crises, or regarded as insignificant (Frank, 1981; Kaufman, 1981).

Here we examine in depth the adjustment that one mildly mentally retarded individual is making to life in the wider community. By utilizing a life history approach, we are able to examine the life of Tim Anthony[1] in some detail, considering not only his life as it is presently lived, but how he reached his current situation. Our study is guided by those points of change which are considered by Tim himself to have been significant and meaningful in his life. We supplement Tim's own reflections on his life with an analysis of the processes by which the changes in his life have taken place. In order to demonstrate how various aspects of his life have played an important role in creating his current life style, we will examine his childhood experiences, treatment by relatives, assistance from the delivery system, and his psychological needs and personal goals.

Tim Anthony is a twenty-four year old, tall, good-looking black man with an I.Q. of 70. Born in Louisiana in February, 1960, he lived there with his unmarried parents and seven siblings until the age of nine, when his mother moved to Los Angeles, taking Tim and several of his siblings with her. They lived in a number of different residential areas in Los Angeles, not merely because Tim's mother frequently moved from one place to another, but also because the children were often placed in foster homes. At the age of seventeen, Tim's mother sent him to the Job Corps in Utah, a residential work "camp" for adolescents from "problem" families. After leaving the Job Corps, Tim spent several months in Los Angeles with his brother and sister-in-law and three to four months at the YMCA, before becoming a participant in an independent living program for mentally retarded individuals. Since his graduation from that program Tim has been living independently, employed in several competitive jobs, and taking classes at a local college.

Tim remembers little about his years in Lousiana. His memories of his father include a happy relationship with him; but he has not seen his father since leaving Los Angeles. Although Tim remembers seven siblings, he is careful to explain that few of them shared the same father, and he is the only one with his father's last name. Tim's mother was married to the father of his oldest sibling. It seems that she never married any of the other fathers. Tim was the only child born in Lousiana, his father's birthplace. The rest of his siblings were born in Texas, the place of his mother's birth. The only other memory Tim has of these early years is an argument the parents had about the paternity of his sister, Chrystal. His mother claimed that Tim's father was also Chrystal's father, but Tim's father denied this.

During his first two years in the Los Angeles area, Tim's mother often moved to various areas of the city, taking the children with her. When Tim was about eleven years old, the mother became "sick" and Tim and his siblings were placed in the first of many foster homes, beginning a pattern of sporadic residences in such homes interspersed with residing with their mother. During this time Tim also started attending Special Education classes, and learned that not only could he not read, but that learning to do so was also problematic.

Tim has many bad memories about this period in his life. His older brother died during a seizure and Tim's other siblings felt that this death had overtones of murder. Supposedly, the brother's father had sold the boy's medication in order to get money. From ages nine through sixteen, two of Tim's siblings and his mother spent time in Camarillo, a state institution for the mentally ill. His mother was labeled schizophrenic. Although Tim denies that his mother ever beat him, he reports that she often beat and abused the other children, using her fists, extension cords, etc. He said she gave his sister a concussion. She stole from Tim and kicked him out of the house. Tim's mother, in turn, was abused by a number of the various men she brought home. One sister and one brother tried to commit suicide.

Tim remembers that he was not without his own negative behaviors. He had a bad temper and he would steal on occasion. Indeed, several of the homes he lived in were designed for maladjusted youths. Finally, because of his potential for violent behavior, at the age of seventeen Tim was sent, against his will, to the Job Corps in Salt Lake city.

After leaving the Job Corps, Tim returned to Los Angeles to live with his younger brother and sister-in-law. After several months Tim became un-happy because he wasn't getting along with his brother and moved into the YMCA for a few months. In the meantime, Tim's brother enrolled him in an independent living skills' training program for mentally retarded individuals. Because he does not consider himself to be retarded, Tim claims that he would never have entered the program had his brother not tricked him. Once enrolled, however, he remained until the time of his graduation.

Tim's childhood, then, was one of poverty; psychological and, most likely, physical abuse; schizophrenic mother and siblings; attempts of suicide by loved ones; criminality; a series of foster homes and residences for the mentally retarded; incarceration in a juvenile detention center; placement againt his will in a Job Corps for wayward youth; and, finally, enrollment in a training program for independent living that had been falsely represented to him. A grim picture and one that would hardly provide even the most optimistic social worker, counselor, or researcher with grounds for predicting, or even hoping, that Tim could make a successful adaptation to life in the community. More reasonable and seemingly more justified predictions would be crime, prison, insanity, institutionalization, anti-social behavior and, at best, a miserable existence on the margins of society. Such predictions would be quite wide of the mark.

Tim has actually adapted quite well to the community. Although he was sent to the Job Corps against his will, he reports that he enjoyed being there for a number of reasons. For the first time in his life he ate three substantial meals a day. He learned about the need for exercise and made it a part of his everyday routine. He acquired a number of independent living skills, from cooking and shopping to cleaning and budgeting. During his stay in the independent living program Tim, in spite of his indignation at being "tricked" into entering it, does report a number of positive experiences. After initially living with two different roommates, each for a brief period of time, Tim began to live entirely on his own. Having learned in the Job Corps the independent living skills provided by the program, Tim often filled his time by attending evening courses at a local college. To get around and to keep physically fit, Tim bought himself a bicycle and rode everywhere. When it broke down, he would fix it himself. On the weekends he would often study, spend time in the local public library, and attend a movie. For most of the three years Tim was a participant in our research, he remained in the independent living program where he was an exemplary citizen. He was never "called on the carpet", and he did everything that was expected of him. Indeed, he was often called upon to assist the staff with other less able or less cooperative clients. By the end of his time in the program, Tim was living alone in a middle class neighborhood in the Los Angeles area, had bought a car, acquired a kitten, and found a job which supplemented his SSI payments.

When new management took over the cafeteria where Tim was employed, he temporarily lost his first job but he soon found another as a short order cook. He has been working at this place for almost a year. He severed one friendship when a friend borrowed his car and wrecked it, putting Tim back on his bicycle. His kitten ran away, but he acquired another one. He continues to see his brother and sister-in-law. He fills his evenings and weekends attending as many classes as his time permits, studying, visiting the local library, and going to movies. His inability to read does not deter Tim from actively pursuing his goals. Budgeting his money well, he never lives beyond his means. He is able to retain his residence in a moderate income neighborhood, and methodically pursues his educational and career goals.

Tim's life, to all outward appearances, is normal and middle class. To be sure, it is not trouble free. Nor is it in all respects "normal", or entirely based on what others might consider to be a firm foundation of a realistic understanding of his capabilities, his limitations, and his potential. Nevertheless, it must be considered a successful life. He is scrupulously moral and he values self-reliance highly. He hopes to improve himself and his position and actively works toward achieving the goals expected in a middle class socio-cultural environment.

Perhaps Kagan's (1978) thesis that less than optimal socialization experiences often can be, and are, overcome has a more general applicability. Tim has certainly overcome a miserable and deprived childhood to reach a level of adaptation that is not often achieved by mentally retarded individuals who have had more supportive backgrounds. But perhaps Tim's adaptation was as much *because* of his background as it was *in spite of it*. It is, on the other hand, also because of certain aspects of Tim's childhood experiences that his adaptation is not as satisfying as it might be.

We have presented a brief chronological record of a number of the events and stages of Tim Anthony's life. This record is only background information and provides little of the flavor of his life. More importantly, it says nothing of the changes that have occurred in Tim himself, those changes as he perceives and interprets them, and as they might be understood in terms of the external conditions and the internal psychological needs that brought them about. In the next section we shall address these themes as we explore the changes that have occurred in Tim's life. Our approach will be to discuss from Tim's own point of view the changes that have taken place in his life and the attitudes, beliefs, and aspirations he now holds. We then add to Tim's account our own understanding of the processes which led to his life as it is currently lived. Following the standards of the life history approach (Crapanzano, 1980; Langness and Frank, 1981; Wilson, 1975), our interpretation of these processes of change and adaptation is based on analyses of the events that Tim, himself, has mentioned, described, and attempted to explain.

The changes that have taken place in Tim's life may be seen as a series of steps that have given him control over his life and his behavior. Indeed, they are viewed this way by Tim himself. Moreover, Tim believes that this control was brought about through his own volition, and through insights he has gained by thinking about himself, and the causes for his behavior. Tim is in his own mind, and to a large degree in fact, a self-made man.

As a child, Tim had practically no control over his chaotic life. His psychotic mother had a succession of men who beat her. Tim reports he hated watching these violent encounters but was powerless to prevent them, just as he was powerless to prevent the beatings his siblings received from their mother. He had a number of operations during his childhood but did not understand, or does not remember, why. He was on special diets, one of which he claims to have consisted of nothing more than one Seven-Up a day. He was given no explanation for these diets. During this time, Tim's mother took him to a psychologist to have his intelligence tested. Tim says she forced him against his will to "play dumb" in order to qualify for Supplemental Security Income. His family moved frequently and he attended at least seven different schools. He had few friends, partly as a result of moving, and partly as a result of rejecting as unsuitable his Special Education classmates. Finally, as mentioned, one of Tim's sisters and one of his brothers attempted suicide during Tim's childhood.

Tim remembers that during these years he felt very alone and the only person he could depend upon was himself. He reports that his childhood was "terrible" and that "things were so bad I just didn't care what happened". He defended himself by having "a heart like a steel wall". His reaction to the chaos and the pain was to repress his feelings and emotions. When a brother died, Tim went into another room and watched television while the rest of the family wept. Later, when they went to view the body, again everyone wept but Tim. He reports that his step-grandmother told him to go back and look at the body. He said to himself "she wants me to cry", but he wouldn't. Looking back on this behavior, Tim seems rather more amazed than remorseful, nevertheless he still describes it as "pretty mean on my part". He talks about those days as if he were a different person as indeed he was.

At eleven, Tim's mother was temporarily placed in a state institution for the mentally ill. Tim and his siblings entered the first of a number of foster homes and institutions. Tim's life between the ages of eleven to seventeen involved a series of moves between foster homes, homes for the mentally retarded, residences with his mother, and twice, placement in a juvenile detention center. This first major change in Tim's life, removal from his mother and family, had a number of consequences. Fortunately, some of the negative consequences were short term while the positive ones established for Tim a pattern of behavior and thinking that has played a large role in his life and still continues today.

Tim describes himself as having had a "bad attitude" during this period of his life. He deeply resented being placed in homes for the mentally retarded. He was accused of stealing and though he does not admit it, it appears that he may have been guilty. At one point his mother took Tim to a psychiatrist who certified him a "kleptomaniac". He had a terrible temper and was in a great number of fights. During these fights, Tim claims to have temporarily "blacked out" and exhibited tremendous strength. As the result of an especially serious fight, Tim's mother took him out of school in the eleventh grade because "she didn't want me hurting nobody else". Tim believes that all the moving from home to home made him mean "cause I was living in so many places by myself. The only person that was there to take care of myself was me. It was terrible too."

It was also at this time, and in these foster homes, that Tim began to be introspective. He attributes this to being temporarily free of the chaos of his family home and from the influence of his mother. He was able to gain perspective, to think about his behavior, and to determine to change it. For the first time he felt he had some control over his life. He began to believe that through self-reflection he could understand it, and through self will he could also change it.

We have only Tim's word for what happened and when it happened, of course. We realize that Tim has reconstructed events and his own understanding of them in the light of changes that took place at later periods in his life. We are reasonably sure, however, that what Tim has told us is his own understanding of what happened. It is, at the very least, what he now believes to have happened. Moreover, what he says makes sense, not only in terms of comments by various counselors and researchers, but also in terms of generally accepted tenets of psychological theory. It is understandable that a young child, removed for the first time in his life from psychotic squalor, should suddenly become aware that life could be different and that one could think about one's life, reflect on one's behavior, and gain some control over it. In addition, it is precisely during this period of puberty and adolescence that an individual's ego identity is believed to be formed (Erikson, 1950). In any case, Tim claims that at this point in his life he became introspective and began to believe that he could think things out and change them. Tim reports that when he was residing with his mother and she was unsuccessfully coping with life,

I said to myself, the funny thing — like I was up to here — talking like a man, or thinking like a man when I'm only so tall and so young. So this is what I said to myself, "Well, when I grow up . . . I help people that wanna help themselves, and that's willing to help themselves. I'm not gonna waste my time tryin' to help nobody that don't wanna help themselves, that's gonna try to make you look like a fool or somethin'." You know?

He has this to say concerning the period between his incarcerations at the juvenile detention center:

I was beginning to get a little wild, but then I calmed my own self down. After getting caught, I told myself that it's not right and so I stopped that.

It would appear from these quotes that Tim had gained some insight at a relatively early age. Consider, however, what he has to say after he had been labeled a kleptomaniac:

I was layin' in the bed . . . I was just thinkin', and this is what I said to myself . . . it just all occurred to my mind. "Stealin' is gonna get me in a lot of trouble. Plus, it's bad anyhow, and I know it's bad. And the only reason I steal is because . . ." I wasn't talking to myself, I was just thinking, I was just layin' there, lookin' straight up at the ceiling, you know. So . . . I was sayin', "This right here, I don't like doin' it. I don't like doin' it for one thing". And then while I was still thinkin', I said, "I don't like doin' it and it can mess me up for quite awhile, and I know it's bad". So about a year later, or just before I turned seventeen, I stopped doin' it.

"So about a year later . . ." makes one a little suspicious. Perhaps he is confused about when things took place. Perhaps he is reinterpreting this particular change in behavior in terms of what he now believes. Perhaps he's attempting to integrate the first instances of this idea with later, more deliberate thoughts on the subject. Regardless of what the uncoverable and real "truth" is, it is clear that Tim now believes that thought and introspection can lead to change and control of one's life. It is also clear that during the next phase of Tim's life, while he was in the Job Corps, more significant and lasting changes took place.

When Tim was seventeen years old and in the eleventh grade, his mother enrolled him in the Job Corps. Though it seems clear, as we indicated above, that she did so because Tim was a behavioral problem and was getting into fights at school, he claims that she was being vicious and took him out of school so that he wouldn't be able to graduate. This interpretation is in perfect accord, as we shall see below, with many of Tim's defenses regarding his limitations, and in particular his inability to read. For Tim, his accomplishments come from within himself, from his thinking, his will, and his power; but his limitations are imposed upon him by outside forces.

Regardless of Tim's ambivalent feelings about leaving school and joining the Job Corps, he enjoyed the time he spent there. Moreover, this period was one of the most significant and influential times of his life, a time when his life changed dramatically, and Tim recognizes this.

Tim was in the Job Corps for eighteen months. During that time he took several training programs including cooking, electronics, and plumbing, as well as a number of academic courses including math, science, and reading. He proudly displays the evaluations and progress reports that he has saved in a notebook from that time. They all contain glowing reports of Tim's progress. It was not the training, however, that he received in these practical matters, though they too had an impact on his life that made this such a significant period, but Tim's realization while in the Job Corps that "I learned that there wasn't nothin' wrong with me, it was my mother, the way she was trying to raise me". It was his family that was "messed up" and not him. He describes the Job Corps itself as "a place for kids with messed up families". In his view, he was there not because of his fighting or stealing, his mental retardation, or his inability to read, but because he was a "kid with a messed up family".

Tim claims that the changes he underwent as the result of this insight were so great they actually changed his physical appearance. He claims that in all the photographs taken of him before he entered the Job Corps he looks so different one would not recognize him. He adds that in these photographs he looked as though he had a lot of problems and that he was disturbed. According to Tim, he acted the way he looked and did so because of living with his family. When a researcher told him that he looked best when he smiles (and he does have a charming smile), he replied that "in the old days I looked like I wanted to fight when I smiled". He reports that when he first went into the Job Corps and tried to talk to "young ladies" they would turn and walk away from him. After six months in the Corps, when he looked at a "young lady", she wanted him to come home with her. He recounts, "I was telling my own self 'I must be gettin' better because people are likin' me' ". He also remembers that during this period he had his first girlfriend, and that this was the first time he had ever cared about anyone.

This was a period, then, when he not only came to believe that what was wrong with him was caused by external forces, his mother and his "messed up" family, but that he could alter his life. He came to believe that he could think about himself, could understand his actions, and, if he wished, could change them. He discovered that as a result of these changes people liked him and he began to care about others. He realized that he could be "normal" and that he enjoyed being so. He has made that his goal and has devoted much of his time and effort, from then until the present, to achieving it . . . or at least, appearing to have achieved it.

Through the good fortune of being taken out of his chaotic home environment and placed in the Job Corps, through his insightfulness and determination, and through his diligence and hard work, Tim has made a successful adaptation to life in the community. He is an ordinary citizen, even a model one. He is also a mentally retarded citizen who cannot read. Tim devotes much time and effort, both physical and psychological, denying to himself and to others that he is retarded, declaring that he has, through his own insight and inner strength, overcome his background and become "normal" in every way. In this he is reminiscent of the de-institutionalized mentally retarded persons described by Edgerton (1967). His rejection of a retarded identity is, in many ways, necessary to his psychological well-being and self-esteem. This denial also contributes, in positive ways, to his successful adjustment to community living. There is a cost, however, not only in the amount of effort the denial takes, but more importantly, in the effect that the form of the denial has upon Tim's social relationships.

Tim often will not admit his inability to read, except of course, when he is powerless to hide it. Tim always denies his label of mental retardation and always provides evidence which supports this denial. His I.Q. of seventy places him just outside the officially defined range of mild mental retardation, defined in terms of I.Q. between 55 and 69. Moreover, Tim is quite adept at superficial interpersonal interaction and his physical appearance is normal, even handsome. Once, when visiting our research offices, he was introduced to a researcher who assumed he was a new member of our research staff. One of the counselors in the independent training program also doubted that Tim was mentally retarded and arranged for a battery of tests and examinations which included I.Q. tests, examinations for neurological impairment and brain damage, and tests for learning disabilities in a number of areas. The results of all this testing simply confirmed that Tim had an I.Q. of 70, showed sporadic hesitation in speech, and could not read. Perhaps more importantly, Tim had been *labeled* mentally retarded, both officially through his mother who had him tested and labeled presumably in order to receive Supplemental Security Income, and through his placement in Special Education classes; and by implication, through his placement in family care homes for the mentally retarded and through his enrollment in the independent living training program. Tim denies that he is mentally retarded and has explana-

tions for anything that makes it appear that he might be. Though he has more
difficulty denying his inability to read (he does on occasion claim to be able
to read now, though admitting that he was not able to in the past), he does
have explanations for this difficulty and is making some small progress in
overcoming it.

According to Tim, any behavior on his part that might make him appear
to be mentally retarded was beyond his control. It was either caused by his
early environment and the people in it, at a time when he had not yet gained
insight and control over his own actions, or he was tricked into it.

We have already presented Tim's claim that his mother forced him to "act
dumb" when being evaluated for eligibility for Supplemental Security Income.
As for his placement in family care homes for the mentally retarded, Tim
claims it was because no other foster home could be found for him and
because he was acting "so wild" during that time. He says he was not acting
normally because *he didn't know how to control himself then*. Thus, his
enrollment in Special Education classes was also the result of his lack of
introspection and self-restraint. In addition, Tim grants that his inability to
read may have contributed to his placement in Special Education classes but
this inability was itself caused by forces outside his control at the time. He
asserts that while in the Job Corps and eating three meals a day he could
learn better and follow what the teachers were telling him. Tim draws all of
this together by attributing his learning difficulties at this stage in his life to
not "eating right" and to his bad attitude, both caused by his family.

As mentioned earlier, Tim feels that he was "tricked" into enrolling in the
independent living training program and blames his brother for it. He reports
that while living at the YMCA and first told about the program he questioned his need for it since, in his opinion, he was already capable of living
on his own. His brother argued that the program would assist with his rent
and would help him find a job. Tim assumed that the clients of the program
would be similar to his peers in the Job Corps who "all graduated from high
school but they didn't have any trade. Or some of them had problems with
their families so they wanted them to get a trade so they could, you know, go
out and find a job". On the basis of this assumption, Tim agreed to visit the
program and, indeed, met a number of normal people whom he assumed
were clients. Actually, they were counselors and family members of potential
clients who were also evaluating the program. Tim claims to have met none
of his fellow clients until he entered the program. He was "tricked" and
remained in the program because he "always finishes anything" he starts.

All of this is simply to explain away circumstantial evidence that might be
misinterpreted by others. There is no doubt in Tim's mind. He knows he is
not mentally retarded and he knows it because, typically, he thought about it.
It was one thing, he says, that he wanted to "figure out" before he was
eighteen (i.e., while he was in the Job Corps): "What I wanted to know for
myself, was I handicapped or what?" He mentions that his father did things

for him when Tim was a child. "If I was somebody retarded, why did my father do that for me? If I was so retarded, why did I go to a public school? So I started thinking about all those things. If I go over here, I must not be retarded. If I could roller skate, ice skate, run, and ride mini-bikes? And have normal friends?" He graduated from the 6th, 7th, and 8th grades with diplomas and how could he do that if he was retarded? No, Tim figured it out, and he was not retarded.

For Tim, there is also a wealth of corroborating evidence. When he was in the family care homes for the mentally retarded he noticed that he was different, that he could think for himself and they couldn't. Moreover, the counselors had to wash and feed some of the other children. Tim could do these things for himself. Many of his fellow clients in the program for independent living are also less capable than Tim and he cites this as further evidence that he is not retarded. He is different from the others. "I'm a tenant but I don't consider myself one of the tenants." He considers himself to be more a member of the program's staff than one of its clients and as evidence points out that he is sometimes asked by the staff to assist with someone less capable than himself, and that he has social relationships with a number of the staff members.

Tim's denial of membership among the mentally retarded and his rejection of his family, the principal reason he is forced to deny mental retardation in the first place, is so complete that in Tim's mind the members of his family inhabit "the fake world" while Time is an inhabitant of "the real world". In the real world a person is trying to make something of himself. For Tim this includes getting a diploma, going to college, and having a normal and successful future life. A person that lives in the fake world is a person that likes to eat, sleep, and occasionally work or go to school but wants "everybody else to take care of him. He's living in his own world. He don't want to be a part of the civilization world." Tim desperately wants to be a part of the "civilization" and "real" world.

Tim's principal handicap, as it is seen by Tim and as it affects his life, is his inability to read. Tim is centrally and continually concerned with it. He believes that his difficulty with reading is his main problem and that if he can overcome this problem he can achieve all his goals including marriage, a college education, and becoming a psychologist.

Although Tim attempts to deal with his illiteracy in some of the same ways that he deals with the label of mental retardation, the fact that he cannot read has more of an impact on his life than does the label. It cannot be attributed to misconceptions of his abilities by others nor can it be totally denied. It is a fact, and as such it has direct and real manifestations and consequences which include being a constant source of threat to Tim's self-esteem. Illiteracy looms large in his life and Tim devotes much time and energy to dealing with it. His efforts include attempts to rationalize it, to overcome it, and to hide it.

Tim's explanations to himself and others for his inability to read overlap with his explanations for being falsely labeled as mentally retarded. They include malnourishment when a student, being moved from school to school, misplacement in Special Education classes, being removed from school by his mother, improper instruction by his brother and so on. Once again, these explanations have to do with forces outside himself over which he had no control at the time and they prominently feature members of his family. It is not Tim's fault, then, that he is unable to read but the fault of circumstance and others.

Since leaving the Job Corps, Tim has continued trying to learn to read. He has been tutored by his brother and has taken a number of courses. Typically his reasons for doing so come from within himself. He has not "learned to read" because, as his mother claimed, the wrath of God would come down on him if he did not, but "I learned to read because *I* wanted to, because of the things I wanted to do". Tim was partly motivated by his brother's observation that college educated women would not marry him if he did not know how to read. He is also motivated, of course, by his desire to be a member of the "real world" and to pursue the goal that symbolizes ultimate success: becoming a psychologist. He tells, poignantly, of an incident in a cooking class when "a young lady" shared her book with him. He pretended to read along with the rest of the class and "I saw all of these people, you know, treating me like I wanted to be treated. And like, they was treating me like the *way that I am*." They were treating him as the real Tim, as a person who, except for unfortunate circumstance, could read.

To hide from others the fact that he has great difficulty in reading, Tim has two basic strategies. He fakes an ability to read as he did in his cooking class and as he does on examinations with predictably disastrous results, or he avoids, when he can, situations in which it might be discovered he cannot read. Often this is done at great personal cost as when he breaks off or avoids relationships with women because he fears they will discover his inability to read and no longer respect him.

So Tim rationalizes, attempts to overcome, and tries to hide his inability to read. In spite of all of this, however, Tim cannot fool himself. He is often discouraged as when he tried to fake his way through an examination in one of his classes. "I was sitting there like I was reading by guessing the words and marking them down. I say, 'Well, this may be right'. I said to myself, 'who am I fooling? I don't know how to read. I shouldn't be in this class.' So in some places it tore me up pretty good. It made me look like the dumbest guy in the world."

But Tim carries on. He has his goal of becoming a psychologist, his desire to be a member of the real world, and his inner resources and strength. In a recent English class the assignment was to read just a few pages a week. Tim proudly reported that he had read thirty one pages in one week and then finished the book in three months. He then finished another in one month.

Tim is sure he will soon become the person he really is and will know how to read like all the other residents of the real world.

As a result of Tim's denial of mental retardation, his occasional denials and constant attempts to conceal his inability to read, and his fear of exposure, his social life has been severely curtailed. This is exacerbated by a continuing need to reject his family and the past that they represent. Finally, the fact that Tim is only minimally intellectually impaired serves to further isolate him. As mentioned earlier, Tim would not associate with his mentally retarded peers in the family care homes, or with those in his Special Education classes. He reports that he would talk to a few of them and was friends with a few for a while until he found out "what kinds of guys they was". Similarly, after he had been "tricked" into entering the training program for independent living and finally met some of the other clients, he says, "I saw all these peoples and I started talking to them like I talked to anybody else, you know. They hardly knew what I was talking about you know. So what I did, I just stopped talking to anybody." Of course, not all the other clients are much more impaired than Tim, but, partly because they are lower functioning and uninteresting to him, and partly because he does not wish to be identified with them, Tim does not interact any more than he must and certainly not as a friend with any of the other clients in the program. Although he socialized with some of the program's staff, these relationships were, for the most part, passing associations. They had occurred because of the situation, and upon Tim's graduation gradually disappeared from his life.

Tim, then, has no real friends among his peers and little contact with persons who are mentally retarded. He chooses not to, both because he has little in common with most of the mentally retarded persons he knows and because he does not want to be identified with them, either by himself or others. Tim, in fact, has no real friends at all. Moreover, it is with women especially that his handicap and his denial of it adversely affect his relationships.

Tim presents himself as attractive to women, especially since his Job Corps days. His stories, however, are confusing and sometimes contradictory. Although, as we mentioned above, Tim reports that the first time he ever really cared about anyone was when he fell in love while in the Job Corps, it is not clear that he has ever had a steady and ongoing romantic relationship with any woman. He had none during the three years that we had research contact with him and when he speaks of the past, with the exception of the instances we discuss below, he tends to speak in generalities and mentions no names or specific details. Indeed, his discussions of women consist primarily of the claim that they are attracted to him and explanations of why he doesn't "mess" with "young ladies".

Tim's earliest reported recollection of involvement with women occurred in the context of being asked whether he had ever had sexual relations with any of the women who were pursuing him. He replied that he had not. He reports that he came close once, when he was about thirteen. He was so tempted that he actually slipped in through a "young lady's" window. Someone came into the room, however, so he had to jump out the window. Tim figures that was a fortunate break because if he had begun to make love at that age he wouldn't have been able to concentrate on his studies or work. He would not, in other words, have been able to lead a life in the "real world" but would have been doomed to live in the "fake world" with guys like his brother who began "messing" with girls at an early age and have been unable to do very well in their studies or work ever since.

Tim reports that while he was in the Job Corps he was "messing" with the wrong young ladies. He knew this because all they wanted was his money. He came across some "that were only looking for a quick lay". He came across others who "were looking for a sucker. Somebody to take care of them for the rest of their life." Tim wasn't fooled, however, and dealt with these women by telling them that he didn't have any money, that he didn't want to get married until he was thirty, and that he didn't want any children. This is the reason, he says, that he never had a regular girlfriend. He reports that these women were either younger than him, or trying to be as smart as him, or they were smarter than him. He figured out what they were doing though so they couldn't have been a whole lot smarter, "or should I say, I wasn't too dumb?"

Whether Tim terminated any relationships he may have had while in the Job corps or whether he women did, and whatever the reason they were ended — or more likely never really established — of a few things we can be reasonably sure. Tim had no long term or satisfactory relationship with a woman while he was in the Job Corps. He fears, at least now and in retrospect, that women will outsmart him and take advantage of him, or that they will not really love and respect him if he is unable to read. Any women with whom he possibly could have established relationships he viewed as unworthy members of the "fake world" who were looking for "someone to take care of them the rest of their life". Those to whom he was attracted were potential threats to his self-esteem as they might reject him because he could not read.

We pointed out that part of Tim's motivation for learning to read resulted from a conversation in which his brother told him that women with college educations would never marry him if he could not read. It is precisely to such women that Tim is attracted as they are members of the "real world" and their acceptance of Tim would validate his denial of any handicap and establish his right to membership in the "real world" also. Indeed, Tim attempted to establish a romantic relationship with a college educated woman, one of the counselors in the independent living training program.

Tim fell in love with his counselor, Martha, and became convinced that she loved him also. Although Martha did not really love Tim, and in fact eventually had him transferred to another counselor because of his infatuation with her, Tim, when questioned by a doubting researcher, could offer all sorts of evidence that proved her romantic interest in him. When asked if Martha had ever actually said she was in love with him, Tim replied that "she said it but then she didn't say it". What she actually said was that she was in love with someone and that she loved him very much, probably in an attempt to discourage Tim's advances. Tim, however, chose to believe that she was speaking of him because of the way she acted toward him. He provides several examples of such behavior. First, she had asked him to dinner, and even though she asked four other tenants to go along, Tim knew that it was really him she was asking because she kept looking at him throughout the meal. She also asked questions that only a girlfriend would ask a boyfriend, for example, how much of a tip you leave at a restaurant. Furthermore, she looked at him in a different way than she looked at the others. This occurred not only in the restaurant but at other times as well. One day when he was sitting on a couch in a class she sat close to him and stared him in the eye. To Tim, this was so blatant a sign of interest in him that he became suspicious. Perhaps she didn't love him after all. Perhaps she was just trying to make him *think* she cared for him. "If you're in a program where you're supposed to have a handicap, but they don't know that you know certain things, certain things that I was there to pick up, then a young lady wouldn't be too interested in you. If she was interested in you, it wasn't because she loved you, it's because she can take you for a sucker. She'd know that you'd never had a girlfriend or somebody that was very friendly or loving to you and she'd be very kind and loving to you. Some young ladies know that they can get — that a guy would take that personally and he would think that she really loved him."

Tim, though he can offer arguments to "prove" that Martha loves him, cannot quite convince himself that a college educated woman could really love him. She was "very sexy and beautiful and smart". She had a Bachelor's Degree and he was in this program for people who are handicapped. He wanted to know why she was interested in him. Was it because she liked him, or because he's good looking, or because he's pretty smart, or because she thinks he's rich because of the clothes he wears? He tested her by telling a lie about having three thousand dollars. He says she tried to find out if he really had that much money and where he kept it, apparently failing the test. To him, her questions simply served to indicate her personal interest in him since that is not something a counselor would ask.

Tim finally "began to realize" that he was twenty and she was twenty-four and too old for him. He "decided" to end the relationship.

His chance to do so came one day when she saw him standing on the street and purposely walked away from him so that he could see her in her tight jeans. He said she was twisting her hips because she knew he was going to look. Now, Tim had already told her that he loved her. He thought to himself that if he looked at her then she'd think that he loved her only for her body. If he ignored her, he figured, then she'd know that he was telling the truth, that he did, in fact, love her. He looked. Master of deceit that he is, "I can make any kind of a person think that I'm a bad guy or a good guy or a selfish no good kind"; his ploy worked. She said, "You see Timothy, me and your love is different". She meant that he only loved her for her body. Or perhaps she meant she only loved him as a friend. Tim isn't sure which, but tends to believe the former.

Tim hasn't seen Martha in a while. He called her occasionally but "it looked like she got tired of hearing the same things" from him and he got tired of hearing "something else" from her. He finally told her that to solve both of their problems they should probably not call each other anymore. She said "bye" and hung up. He decided not to make a fool of himself and call her again. He said he stuck to his "manhood" and didn't call her.

Tim, then, is not attracted to women who may be attracted to him. He most certainly will have nothing to do with fellow "tenants" in the training program for independent living. When one of the women in the program asked Tim if he would like to see her do a strip-tease, and removed her blouse and bra when he jokingly answered in the affirmative, Tim beat a hasty retreat. Tim would be endangering his denial of being handicapped if he established a relationship with a handicapped woman. Rather, to validate his denial of a handicap and his claim to a rightful place in the "real world", Tim must attempt to establish a relationship with someone who is clearly in the "real world": someone educated, smart, and sexy, like Martha. Since such relationships don't really happen, Tim must manufacture evidence that they do by misinterpreting the behavior of the women in whom he is interested. The evidence wears thin, even for Tim. He becomes suspicious, has doubts, and then "ends" the "relationship". He repeated this behavior with his next female counselor, who, according to Tim, constantly and deliberately was sexually provocative with him. He was transferred to a male counselor before he could actually declare his love.

Tim tells us that in the past he chose not to associate with mentally retarded persons at all. During the time we worked with him, this was also generally true. As mentioned earlier he did have the one friend, but quickly abandoned him when he wrecked Tim's car. He also attended some of the group activities of the independent living program. But generally, during our contact with him, Tim was pretty much a loner. His main contacts were with a brother and sister-in-law who lived nearby and with the researcher who worked with him. In fact, this may in part have been the reason for the success of the research with Tim. He was willing to spend long periods of time talking about himself to a reseacher because he had no one else to talk to.

It was well into the research before it was discovered that Tim was seeing his brother, and even later before it was discovered that their current relationship is an amicable one. Tim portrayed his brother as someone who took advantage of him by misappropriating his money when he left the Job Corps; is a "player"; smokes marijuana; cheats on his wife and beats her; insults Tim by calling him retarded; and on and on. It was only discovered by accident that this same brother often had Tim over for dinner; that they celebrated a number of holidays together including Tim's birthday; that the brother frequently invited Tim to play handball; that the brother had arranged a joint long-distance telephone call to their mother; and so on. Tim failed to straightforwardly offer any of this information. The genial nature of Tim's relationship with his brother was only discovered by the researcher's dogged pursuit of inadvertent mentions of the incidents.

For some reason, Tim did not want it known that the relationship with his brother had become more harmonious or that his brother had any redeeming qualities at all. As we have pointed out, Tim's coping strategies and his maintenance of self-esteem rest in part on his rejection of his background and his family. They reside in the "fake world" of those who do nothing to help themselves and who do not strive to succeed. Tim blames them for his problems and disassociates himself from them and from their way of life. Yet Tim is lonely. His brother offers company and kindness and Tim accepts. This relationship does not fit with Tim's construction of reality, with his attribution of blame for his problems, so he denies that it exists, at least to the researcher, if not to himself. Tim claims that he has "turned out better" than anyone else in his family. His constant criticism of his brother's life style may be seen as an attempt to make himself and his life look better by comparison.

For Tim, the dichotomy between the fake and the real worlds is the important one in evaluating individuals. He rejects a classification of normal and mentally retarded people or of literate and illiterate individuals. Tim recognizes the existence and social importance of these other dichotomous views of the world of course, and, as we have shown, devotes a good deal of effort to denying or concealing the way they have been applied to him. In his own mind, however, the important distinction is the one between the real world and the fake world. The principal dimension that distinguishes residents of the real world from those in the fake world is the individual's attempt to help and improve himself. There are, of course, positive consequences of trying to help one's self, but in Tim's mind it is the trying itself that distinguishes people who are worthwhile from those who are not.

Tim, himself, goes at self-improvement with a vengeance. His days are literally filled with work and school; to the extent that it was difficult at times in the course of the research to make an appointment with him. He does not watch television as it "wastes time and it makes you stop thinking". And as we have seen, thinking is centrally important in helping one's self. For Tim, insight and understanding are the necessary preconditions for self-improvement. He interprets his past life course as a series of changes which followed insights into his attitudes, behavior, and beliefs. These insights came as Tim was progressively freed from the chaos of his childhood with his family. The greatest change, not surprisingly, came during his adolescence in the Job Corps. There Tim adopted the attitudes and set the course that he follows to this day. Pushed by his insight, his will, and his resolve, and drawn toward his goal of becoming a psychologist, Tim has created a life in the real world. He sees himself as capable and always learning. He goes to school and aspires to learn to read. He has a job, an apartment, and a pet. He has "adopted" a child by giving regularly to a charity. He wants to marry, have children, and be a contributing member of society. To be sure, there is a cost to his denial of any handicap, particularly in his social relationships, but all in all, Tim has made an admirable adjustment by any standard. Most importantly, however, he has succeeded by his own standards and through his own efforts. He has achieved and continually strives to maintain his place in the real world.

ACKNOWLEDGEMENT

This research was supported by grant NIE-G-80-0016 from the National Institute of Education and grant NICHD HD 11944-02 from the National Institute of Child Health and Human Development. We wish to thank Dr. Claudia Mitchell-Kernan, Dr. Sharon Sabsay, and Dr. Belinda Tucker for their supervision of the data collection. We also wish to thank Marsha Bollinger who collected the data and provided many insightful comments and suggestions.

NOTE

1. See Koegel (1984) for a brief description of Tim.

REFERENCES

Buhler, C. and F. Massarik (eds.)
    1968 *The course of human life: A study of goals in the humanistic perspective.* New York: Springer.
Crapanzano, V.
    1980 *Tuhami: Portrait of a Moroccan.* Chicago: University of Chicago Press.
Dailey, C. A.
    1971 *Assessment of lives: Personality evaluation in a bureaucratic society.* San Francisco: Jossey-Bass.
Edgerton, R. B.
    1967 *The cloak of competence: Stigma in the lives of the mentally retarded.* Los Angeles: University of California Press.
Edgerton, R. B.
    1983 Failure in community adaptation: The relativity of assessment. *In* K. T. Kernan, M. J. Begab and R. B. Edgerton (eds.), *Environments and behavior: The adaptation of mentally retarded persons* (pp. 123—143). Baltimore, MD: University Park Press.
Edgerton, R. B.
    1984 Introduction. *In* R. B. Edgerton (ed.), *Lives in process: Mildly retarded adults in a large city* (pp. 1—7). Washington, D.C.: American Association on Mental Deficiency, Monograph Number 6.

Erikson, E. H.
   1963 *Childhood and society*, Second Edition. New York: W. W. Norton and Co., Inc.
Erikson, E. H.
   1975. *Life history and the historical moment*. New York: W. W. Norton and Co., Inc.
Frank, G.
   1981 *Venus on wheels: The life history of a congenital amputee*. Doctoral Dissertation. Department of Anthropology, University of California, Los Angeles.
Hughes, C. C.
   1974 *Eskimo boyhood: An autobiography in psychosocial perspective*. Lexington: University Press of Kentucky.
Kagan, J.
   1978 The baby's elastic mind. *Human Nature, 1:* 66—73.
Kaufman, S.
   1981 Cultural components of identity in old age: A case study. *Ethos, 9*(1): 51—87.
Kennan, K.
   1984 *Time in her life: A Down's woman's personal account*. Doctoral Dissertation. Department of Anthropology, University of California, Los Angeles.
Kennedy, J. G.
   1977 *Struggle for change in a Nubian community: An individual in society and history*. Palo Alto: Mayfield Publishing.
Kernan, K. T. and P. Koegel
   1984 Employment experiences of community-based mildly retarded adults. *In* R. B. Edgerton (ed.), *Lives in process: Mildly retarded adults in a large city* (pp. 9—26). Washington, D.C.: American Association on Mental Deficiency, Monograph Number 6.
Koegel, P.
   1984 Black "six-hour retarded children" as young adults. *In* R. B. Edgerton (ed.), *Lives in process: Mildly retarded adults in a large city* (pp. 145—171). Washington, D.C.: American Association on Mental Deficiency, Monograph Number 6.
Kuper, H.
   1978 *Sobhuza II, Ngwenyama and King of Swaziland: The story of an hereditary ruler and his country*. New York: Africana Publishing Company.
Langness, L. L. and G. Frank
   1981 *Lives: An anthropological approach to biography*. Novato, California: Chandler and Sharp Publishers, Inc.
Mandelbaum, D. G.
   1973 The study of life history: Gandhi. *Current Anthropology, 14*(3): 177—206.
Mintz, S. W.
   1974 *Worker in the cane: A Puerto Rican life history*. New York: W. W. Norton and Co., Inc.
Riegel, K. F.
   1974 Adult life crises: A dialectic interpretation of development. *In* N. Datan and L. H. Ginsberg (eds.), *Life-span development psychology: Normative life crises*. New York: Academic Press.
Wilson, P. J.
   1975 *Oscar: An inquiry into the nature of sanity*. New York: Vintage Books.

ROBERT B. EDGERTON

A CASE OF DELABELING: SOME PRACTICAL AND THEORETICAL IMPLICATIONS

One of the phenomena associated with deinstitutionalization is the official delabeling of persons previously labeled "mentally retarded". Delabeling commonly occurs when someone previously diagnosed, labeled and sometimes receiving services as a mentally retarded person, seeks new or additional services from some component of the mental retardation community service delivery system. When such a person is evaluated, or reevaluated, by a Regional Center or another agency and is found to have an I.Q. above that required for eligibility, the label "mentally retarded" may be replaced by another, such as "schizophrenic" or "learning handicapped" or the label may simply be expunged and the erstwhile mentally retarded person may be declared to be of borderline or average intelligence. As a result of this process of delabeling, and contrary to established belief, a person may be mentally retarded one day and not mentally retarded the next.

Delabeling has received little systematic study, yet its consequences have profound practical implications for the lives of delabeled persons. Delabeling also has relevance for theories concerning the effects of labeling. By examining this process, we shall attempt to show that a person who is labeled mentally retarded may be subjected to a concerted process of socialization that reduces his competence, not only while the label is applied to him but long after it has been removed.

THEORETICAL BACKGROUND

It has long been argued in the social sciences that persons who are stereotyped, tagged or labeled as deviant or undesirable may come to alter their behavior as if a self-fulfilling prophecy were at work. Frank Tannenbaum (1938: 19–20) provided one of the earliest formulations of this perspective when he wrote that by arresting juvenile offenders society made them what they were described as being; "The process of making the criminal, therefore, is a process of tagging, defining, identifying, segregating, describing, emphasizing, making conscious and self-conscious; it becomes a way of stimulating, suggesting, emphasizing, and evoking the very traits complained of". Two decades later, Lewis A. Dexter (1956; 1958) extended this perspective to the mentally retarded, insisting that they were similarly transformed by a process of social labeling.

This perspective has come to be known as "societal reaction theory", and it has grown in sophistication and influence. Whether conceived of in terms of "labeling" or "attribution", this perspective has asserted that persons whom

101

society designates as deviant or undesirable are likely to take on roles that
are consistent with that designation (Lemert, 1951). The tempting simplicity
of the perspective and its common-sense appeal have led to an outpouring of
conceptual refinements and empirical applications, but there is still widespread debate over how best to conceptualize the process by which labels are
thought to produce self-fulfilling outcomes, and indeed, over whether there is
any satisfactory evidence that labels actually produce such effects (Sagarin,
1975).

Since the mid 1950s when Dexter wrote, debate concerning the effects of
labeling the mentally retarded has intensified. Much of the controversy has
centered around labeling in the school system. The sensational assertions
about the effects of teacher expectancies on student performance by
Rosenthal and Jacobsen in their book, *Pygmalion in the Classroom* (1968),
influenced many investigators. The later work of Mercer (1970; 1973) was
also influential. The concept of the "6-hour retarded child" was one result.
"Mainstreaming" was another. The effects of classification and labeling on
community adaptation have also been examined and debated (MacMillan,
Jones and Aloia, 1974; Hobbs, 1975). Critical reviews of the research
literature on the effects of labeling mentally retarded persons have led to a
number of conclusions. These reviews agree that while the label "mentally
retarded" is typically avoided as being stigmatizing, the effects of this label on
the self-esteem or social competence of labeled persons have not been clearly
demonstrated (Yoshida, 1974; Dusek, 1975; MacMillan, 1977; Guskin,
1978; Rowitz, 1981).

These reviewers, and others, point out that most research on the effects of
the label, mental retardation, have greatly over-simplified what is a highly
complex, non-linear, interactive process. More specifically, this research has
inadequately considered the pre-labeling experiences that may have produced low self-esteem and social incompetence prior to the imposition of any
label. Moreover, the possible presence and salience of more than one
stigmatizing label, and more than one labeler is too seldom documented,
especially in regard to setting-specific research such as that characteristically
done in schools. Neither have the predicted effects of labeling usually been
clearly specified, nor have the direct or indirect means by which these effects
are brought about been adequately detailed or controlled. The duration of
the presumed effects has been as little studied as the mechanisms that are
presumed to maintain them. Finally, research that continuously examines the
effects of the process of labeling in the totality of a person's life experiences
over a substantial period of time is altogether lacking.

THE RESEARCH BACKGROUND

Over the past decade, members of the Socio-Behavioral Research Group of
the Mental Retardation Research Center at the University of California, Los

Angeles,[1] have utilized a variety of naturalistic, ethnographic research procedures to study the community adaptation of mentally retarded adults over extended periods of time. As described elsewhere (Edgerton and Langness, 1978), we have utilized a variety of data elicitation techniques in addition to the unobtrusive participant-observation that is the basis of ethnography. We accompany and observe mentally retarded persons in all of the public — and some of the private — activities that make up their everyday lives. We interview all persons (friends, spouses, co-workers, siblings, parents, caretakers, social workers, and the like) whose beliefs, attitudes, or behavior appear to be relevant. We also seek out available documents such as medical records, or test results. Often we follow the persons in our research sample for several years.

The data that we assemble by these various procedures are numerous, complex and sometimes contradictory. Efforts to reduce these qualitative data to simple, linear, cause and effect inferences such as assertions about the effects of labeling, are usually very difficult, if not impossible. Thus, despite the unique richness of our data relating to labeling processes in the lives of mentally retarded persons living in community settings, we can seldom point to direct cause and effect relationships. That is so for all the reasons previously mentioned. it is also so because we cannot fail to see clearly the complex, ambiguous and ever-changing character of the lives these people lead; these lives are a kaleidoscopic product of intellectual abilities, past experiences, current interactions, goals, fears and aspirations — and all those other factors that influence human behavior. In this complex world it is ordinarily impossible to identify labeling as an event or process that causes, or even necessarily conduces toward, such outcomes as low self-esteem or diminished social competence. All we can say with assurance is that the mentally retarded persons in our research samples regard the label, mental retardation, as highly discrediting, and attempt to avoid having it applied to them. But we cannot say what the effects may be when any of the many possible labelers applies some version of the label to someone in our samples. How information about such a label as "slow", "slow learner", "brain damaged", "educationally handicapped" or even "mentally retarded" is actually conveyed to the labeled person, and how that person comprehends the information is a complex interchange in its own right. The ways in which interchanges of information about the label occur over years is still more complex. To assume, then, that all persons labeled mentally retarded, or even that all persons receiving services from a Regional Center as a mentally retarded person, will be affected in comparable ways is simplistic.

Instead of concentrating on labels and their putative effects, we wish to call attention to processes of socialization within the community care system which routinely serve to teach "mentally retarded" persons to be incompetent *even* when these persons either do not know they have been labeled mentally retarded, or when they largely or entirely reject the label. These processes or "socialization for incompetence" consist of the expectations and practices of parents, peers, residential caretakers, workshop employees, Regional Center counselors, social workers and others who in their aggregate make up the effective "community" and sub-culture for persons who are receiving services from the Regional Center system. Briefly, these processes of socialization include expectations and practices that: (1) systematically restrict access to normal experiences, and, (2) produce and reinforce dependent, inappropriate and incompetent attitudes and behavior. Some of these restrictions and practices are coercively enforced, others involve active or passive collaboration on the part of the "mentally retarded" person.

The presence and impact of such processes has often been noted in "total institutions" such as mental hospitals (Goffman, 1961). It has also been asserted that such effects can occur even when the persons involved are not residents of large institutions, but are only the recipients of outpatient therapy and rehabilitation. For example, Scott (1969: 119) has written that:

When those who have been screened into blindness agencies enter them, they may not be able to see at all or they may have serious difficulties with their vision. When they have been rehabilitated, they are all blind men. They have learned the attitudes and behavior patterns that professional blindness workers believe blind people should have. In the intensive face-to-face relationships between blindness workers and clients that make up the rehabilitation process, the blind person is rewarded for adopting a view of himself that is consistent with his rehabilitators' view of him and punished for clinging to other self-descriptions ... Indeed, passage through the blindness system is determined in part by his willingness to adopt the experts' view about self.

Passage through the mental retardation system appears to have equivalent consequences for mentally retarded persons, yet the effects of this system have apparently not been demonstrated in the same way that they have for large institutions (Zigler and Balla, 1977; Bercovici, 1980). We believe that compelling evidence for the assertion that the mental retardation system produces social incompetence — just as the blindness system produces blindness — is provided by the lives of persons who were subjected to the expectations and practices of this system for many years before they were found to have average or above average intelligence and were consequently delabeled.

DELABELING

It has been known for many years that some persons who have been found to have low I.Q.'s and have been institutionalized as a result, were later — often *much* later — found to possess I.Q.'s that were average or better. Deafness, emotional trauma, cultural difference and other factors have been implicated in the I.Q. test "errors". Some of these anecdotes have achieved considerable notoriety as in the case of Joey (Deacon, 1971), and Larry, the subject of a recent CBS television drama (McQueen, 1973). More recently, Klemke and

Tiedemann (1981) have discussed the theoretical significance of studying the "falsely accused" deviant, a point made earlier by Becker (1963).

Mistakes in labeling or "false accusations" of deviance are undeniably tragic, yet the impression persists that they are infrequent. Our research indicates that mistakes in labeling the mildly retarded and subsequent delabeling are sufficiently common events to constitute a significant issue for mental retardation service delivery system personnel. For example, although precise records were not available, counselors at two Regional Centers in Los Angeles estimated that these two centers alone probably "closed the cases", i.e., delabeled, at least 50 mildly retarded clients during 1980.[2] In our own research, it was found that in a cohort of 48 mildly retarded adults whom we studied from 1976 through 1978, 8 were delabeled when they were reevaluated by a Regional Center and found to have I.Q.'s well above 70. One of these cases of delabeling has been reported by Turner (1980).

THE EFFECTS OF DELABELING

Our research indicates that most persons who are delabeled do not respond to this change in labeled status with visibly more competent or independent behavior, even though rapid improvement is often anticipated by the service system personnel who participate in the delabeling process. There are many reasons why it is not possible to attribute the failure of "mentally retarded" persons who are delabeled to make rapid improvement in social competence, independence or other aspects of adaptive behavior solely to their past experience of being "socialized for incompetence". Most of these persons are delabeled in the context of complex social or personal upheaval. In some instances, a person may have been hospitalized as a result of suicide attempt or bizarre behavior. Hospitalization often affects the person's residential arrangement, work status and network of friends and relatives. Thus while such an episode may lead to reevaluation and the discovery that the formerly retarded person has a borderline or average I.Q., the newly delabeled person typically faces a radically different set of social and psychological demands — to find a new place to live, to renegotiate eligibility for SSI as a mentally ill rather than mentally retarded person, to reestablish social ties and friendships in a new neighborhood, and so on. When such persons fail to display improved adaptive behavior — and they do fail — the reason for the failure cannot reasonably be located solely in past socialization experiences. Present circumstances, including psychological and emotional trauma, must also play a determinative role.

It is only when the persons who are delabeled are free of acute emotional distress, and when their social arrangements are undisturbed, that it is possible to examine the part that past socialization for incompetence plays in their efforts to shed the role of "mentally retarded person". While any case of delabeling is necessarily accompanied by contaminating circumstances that complicate analysis, the following case is relatively free of contamination, and serves to illustrate the processes of socialization for incompetence to which I have referred.

JOHN MILLON

John R. Millon had first been labeled "brain damaged" when he was four years old. In the summer of 1973, when he was 21 years old, John was living in Vista House, a large group home, in Southern California where he was receiving S.S.I. benefits as a "mentally retarded" man with "permanent brain damage". After two routine I.Q. testing sessions had indicated that John was *not* mentally retarded he was referred to a third psychological clinic for evaluation. John introduced himself to the clinical psychologist who was to "test him out" by volunteering that he was "brain damaged". However, following a battery of tests, including various personality inventories and the WAIS, the psychologist concluded that "there was no evidence of such damage". Instead he reported of John that, "He can be fairly productive, creative and innovative". His I.Q., full scale, was 102. John and the mental retardation delivery system personnel were informed of these findings. Overnight, John officially shed his retarded label of 17 years standing — he was "delabeled". Shedding the *role* of a mentally retarded person was not so easily accomplished.

In what follows, I shall first sketch the outlines of John's life, especially the labels that were applied to him, and the role expectations that various persons had of him. Next I shall describe his perceptions of his life, including his delabeling and his efforts to "become normal". The result is a very partial life history at best. It is more a vignette drawn from every available source. For the early parts of John's life, various documents and the remembrances of others are used. For later years our own observations of John's behavior, and the perspectives of others who knew him were used to supplement his own accounts.

JOHN'S LIFE BEFORE DELABELING

John's adoptive parents, Audrey and Ralph, lived in a modest 2-bedroom house in a low-middle income neighborhood in a medium-sized city to the east of Los Angeles. When Ralph, a salesman, and Audrey, a registered nurse, were unable to have children after 10 years of marriage, they adopted John who was then 4. In Audrey's recollection, he was never normal. She insists that she knew from the first that he was neurologically handicapped and she suspected that he was a victim of permanent brain damage. He seemed agitated and uncoordinated, with speech that was slow to develop and slurred. To her he was "certainly" not normal. Audrey sought comfort from her Seventh Day Adventist Church, and from the nurses and doctors at the local community hospital where she worked. Audrey says that a doctor at this hospital diagnosed John as "brain damaged", but apparently, she got little help, for the most part being told to "love John" and to have another child "of her own". At this time, in 1956, there were few services available for John and he appears to have received nothing beyond infrequent pediatric care. In any event, no medical records are available concerning John's physical condition before he entered school.

School records, too, are scanty, but a teacher who remembered John recalled that Audrey told everyone at the school that John was brain damaged and could not be expected to learn at a normal pace. This teacher recalled that John was thought of, at least by some teachers, as a "neurologically handicapped, slow learning" child, but how common these expectancies were and how they may have been conveyed to John is difficult to say. John, himself, recalls that the teachers recognized him to be a "slow" student, but that they blamed his mother for creating this situation by her incessant overprotection and deprecation of him. There is no confirmation of this. We do know that John was in regular classes and that his mother helped him with his homework. Despite poor grades, he was promoted from grade to grade on schedule.

There is little reliable evidence concerning his early home environment. John recalls his adopted father as being meticulous, distant but kindly, and Audrey as domineering, critical and overprotective. John still dwells on toys which were given to him by his biological mother before her death, saying that Audrey often tried to throw these toys away but that he always managed to retrieve them. He can remember that Audrey often said that she loved him, but he never felt any love from her, not even affection. John felt more affection from his father but seldom had anything to do with him.

It is clear that John's contacts with other children were very carefully regulated. Audrey chose his friends, apparently restricting them to children with some kind of physical handicap. John was not allowed to ride a bike, engage in ordinary games or sports, or choose his own friends to come over to the house. Audrey took him to and from school, and on weekend outings. She remembers him in these pre-adolescent years as uncoordinated, nervous, easily upset, and in need of her constant protection, however much this placed a burden on her and her marriage. To her, John was a burden and an obligation; she rejects any suggestion that she "over-protected" him. He needed her protection and she gave it. So it was until John was thirteen. As John became a teenager, he became increasingly difficult to supervise and control. We know from the reports of physicians and social workers that Audrey repeatedly sought help from friends and agencies because she felt John becoming more and more hostile and beyond her control. For one thing, John now insisted on having friends of his own. His parents were certain that these young people would lead the "suggestible" John into all sorts of trouble. Some trouble had already occurred, it seems, since John was said to have startled and frightened several families in the neighborhood by entering their houses uninvited. He was also said to have stolen money from his parents. Some of the reports by physicians about Audrey and Ralph at this time refer to them as being in "despair" about John and "inept" in their efforts to cope with him. In November of 1966, Audrey took John to a child psychiatrist.

Six months later, when John was 15, the first officially recognized crisis in his life took place. John was charged by the police with stealing women's underclothes. A juvenile court hearing concluded that he was "in danger of leading a desolute (*sic*) life", but took no further action. Three months later he was arrested while he was looking through the window of a neighbor's bedroom at a teenaged girl who was dressing herself. The blinds were not drawn and it was not difficult for John to stand outside the window, unseen from the street. John was held at Juvenile Hall until a subsequent juvenile court proceeding declared him a ward of the court and sent him to *Boy's Haven*, a home for delinquent boys. The court heard testimony from the child psychiatrist who had been seeing him since November of the previous year, to the effect that John was "mentally retarded and brain damaged", although no I.Q. test score was reported. He was also declared to be a "sexual psychopath". The psychiatrist also wrote to the court about Audrey's role in John's "problem":

Much sexual preoccupation came to the fore. It quickly became clear that this was an area where his father could or would not talk with him at all and one in which his mother felt very uncomfortable. They rather obviously wished the whole concern would sort of 'go away'. His mother tried extremely hard to cope with this problem and all other problems and felt she was getting no help from his father at all. She tended strongly to keep concerned with areas more appropriate to be concerned with in a much younger boy.

John's troubles continued in Boy's Haven, the home for delinquent boys. He was accused of stealing from other boys, of frequent enuresis, and of unacceptable personal hygiene. As John's difficulties mounted so did Audrey's anxieties. She arranged through the probation department for him to be admitted as an inpatient at a nearby hospital where he underwent neurological tests for 7 days. Audrey says that he was diagnosed as suffering "permanent brain damage", but no record of the examiner's report seems to have survived.

After John had been at Boy's Haven for almost 3 years, Audrey received approval of the probation department for another neurological examination. The neurologist reported that John was "alert" and "oriented" but that, "His affect, however, is flat. In general his responses seem more appropriate for a child of eight or ten years . . . the patient rarely gave any answer without looking to his mother for approval." No thought disorder was found, nor any significant neurological impairment. The neurological report concluded as follows:

It is the opinion of this examiner that this patient has a severe character disorder and that prognosis for the achievement of a state of responsible self-support is very unlikely. He will soon be eligible for the draft. It would appear that he would be a complete misfit in any of the services.

After John had lived in Boy's Haven for 3 years, the director of social services, a psychiatric social worker who was familiar with John throughout his stay there, wrote to John's juvenile probation officer in 1970 to request a new placement. This report concluded that John could progress no further in Boy's Haven and urged that John be sent to another facility out of the reach of his mother.

A great deal of (John's) lack of growth comes, it would appear, from interaction with his family. He has frequent visits from them and seems to regress as a result. This, it seems, comes from his mother's insistence that he is neurologically *handicapped* (and I underline "handicapped") and therefore inadequate and uncapable (*sic*). This vision of his personal efficacy seems to be internalized by (John) as it is his learned habit, over a life time of experience, to meet his affectual needs. This social worker's firm belief is that (John) is *not*, I repeat, is *not* neurologically handicapped in any broad, general sense of the phrase. He may have minimal neurological damage but he consistently manages to sink baskets from all over the court no matter who or how many of his peers (or staff for that matter) are guarding him. And although he speaks slowly and hesitantly, he shows good thought and gives extremely logical solutions to group problems.

The report concluded by saying that, "Briefly, (John) is a boy capable of making it in this world but only if he is given some fresh and *fair* challenges unincumbered (*sic*) by those who would define him as incapable".

There is no record of what probation department officials made of the discrepancy between this report and the others, but we do know that shortly after the social worker's report was submitted, John was sent to live with relatives in a rural area in Oregon where he spent six months and graduated from high school at the age of 19. John was now released from probation. It is not apparent why John did not remain longer in Oregon, but just prior to his graduation, Audrey applied for Aid to the Disabled (ATD) in Southern California, saying that John could return from Oregon if arrangements were made for him to move directly to a family care facility. In the summer of 1971, ATD was approved and John was placed in a family care home, and assigned to a sheltered workshop for vocational training.

The reports justifying these placements and the granting of ATD ignore the Boy's Haven social worker's report and continue to describe John as mentally retarded and in need of close supervision. For example, an ATD report dated July 27, 1971 concluded that "As reported from Mrs. (Millon) and the other reports we received (John) functions on a mildly retarded level with many behavior problems . . . Because of his bizarre behavior (John) is an extremely difficult boy to place. He would frighten many people because of his size (John was then 6' 2½ and 151 lbs.) and his bizarre actions. Supervision has to be close and firm."

Another ATD report at the same time described John as living with "five other mentally retarded boys". John was described as follows: "Client walks awkwardly and speech is slurred. Speaks slowly as if he is trying to assemble thoughts. Caretaker states he still wets bed, is domineering and aggressive." The report did not note that John had only been under the caretaker's supervision for 4 days when this evaluation was made, nor did it comment on the fact that John was then taking 5 mg. of Valium three times a day, and 8 mg. of Chlortrimeton (for an allergy) three times a day.

Three months later, John was examined by a physician, who wrote that the "diagnosis" was "mental retardation" and the "prognosis" was "poor — patient is not employable because of mental retardation". The documents approving the award of ATD also include a report from a licensed psychologist who had 3 one hour interviews with John. The psychologist's report recommended granting ATD based on John's anxieties, confusions and poorly formed identity. But the report stressed that John was not "anti-social" and that, although no testing was done, John's "intellectual capacity is probably within the average range of intelligence".

If this psychological assessment was taken seriously, it did not find its way into John's diagnosis. He remained "mentally retarded". Neither is there any indication that John was told of this evaluation of his intelligence; he denies being told, and the ATD records show that when he was interviewed by an ATD eligibility worker a few days after the psychologist's report was filed, he answered a question about the cause of his handicap by saying that he was "permanently brain damaged". It should also be noted that if John ever took an I.Q. test, there was no record of it at this time.

During the next two years, John moved from the first family care home to a second. Reports by both family caretakers refer to his inability to manage even simple self-maintenance tasks, they also emphasize his emotional immaturity. Indeed, his second caretaker requested "stronger medication" for him and an obliging physician prescribed Mellaril (Thioridazine), 30 mg., three times a day. The possible effects of this anti-psychotic drug on his adaptation are nowhere recorded. Throughout this period John worked at a sheltered workshop where he performed simple and routine tasks. He complained about the monotony of the work and the low pay but his relationships with other workshop clients and staff were apparently congenial. In both settings — family care and the workship — John was seen as a mentally retarded person, one who was dependent on others for supervision and for help with most of the routine demands of life.

As a client of a Regional Center, John's file came up for routine review in April 1973. On April 11, 1973, a licensed clinical psychologist administered the WAIS to him. His full-scale I.Q. was found to be 94. He was also given the Vineland Social Maturity Scale and the Bender Visual Motor Gestalt Test. The psychologist's conclusion was that, "He was pleasant and communicated well during testing using a vocabulary on the average normal level". A few days later the Regional Center assigned another licensed psychologist to evaluate John's intelligence. In addition to the Bender, John was given the Raven Progressive Matrices Test. The results were reports as follows: "Here the client scores near the 75th percentile compared with his age peers. This indicates an estimated I.Q. of 110 or within the bright normal classification. It indicates the client to have sufficient reasoning ability to pursue a semi-professional to professional occupation." John was not informed of the results of these tests. Instead, he was moved to Vista House, a large board and care facility which offered its residents considerable independence.

When the director of Vista House was sent these test results, she requested that John be referred to a third clinical psychologist. John visited this clinic on June 20, 1973, and, as mentioned before, introduced himself as "brain damaged". It was from this evaluation that John was found to have a WAIS full-scale I.Q. of 102. When this result, along with the previous two evaluations, reached the Regional Center, they "closed" John's case on the grounds that his "high" I.Q. and his "high level of functioning at Vista House" made it clear that he was not developmentally disabled. As far as the Regional Center was concerned, John was no longer mentally retarded. He was officially delabeled.

JOHN'S REACTION TO DELABELING

When John was told that he was not mentally retarded, he reacted with elation and confusion. He immediately called his mother with the news. She refused to discuss the matter and hung up the telephone. He discussed his new status — that of a "normal" person — with the staff at Vista House. Since he was still receiving Supplemental Security Income (S.S.I.), replacing A.T.D., as an "occupationally handicapped person", he remained under the supervision of a social worker and a rehabilitation counselor. They agreed that he should remain at Vista House until he could make the transition to competitive employment and independent living. A target date of January 1, 1974 was agreed upon as a conservative time-table, one that John should have no difficulty meeting. In the meantime, John was to work at Vista House as a janitor (for $48 a month) and was to have greatly increased freedom, including the right to go and come as he pleased.

For the first time in his life John was an employee, not a client, and he was free to stay out at night. John's efforts to take on his new freedoms and responsibilities lasted only 2 weeks. At that point he announced that he "wanted freedom but wanted it regulated" and put himself "on restriction" a category used for clients at Vista who are denied the right to leave their rooms after dinner. During this initial transitional period John failed miserably at his work duties, neglecting his janitorial chores most of the time in favor of his self-appointed role as "counselor" to other clients. Not only did he neglect his job, he imposed his counseling on unwilling clients — and staff as well — becoming abusive to them when they objected. He loudly and haughtily told one and all that he had been tested and had been found superior to all of them. In fact, he did not know what his newly tested I.Q. was, and variously reported it as anything from 85 to 210, sometimes saying that 85 was the "highest" he had scored.

When he was first delabeled, he took immediate advantage of his freedom to stay out nights, going to movies and bars. He apparently drank alcohol and smoked marijuana on these evenings and may have had sexual experiences, including homosexual ones. He had never been free to use the telephone before and now he did so extravagantly, charging long distance calls to various numbers including Audrey's. When John was asked why he put himself on restriction he answered this way:

I felt that I just couldn't handle it, like I had problems you know, drug-wise, able to handle myself, acceptable, which I wasn't. I just felt guilty, that . . . that . . . was it for me? You know . . . I think I just didn't want to face reality or something.

(What was the reality you didn't want to face?) That I was *normal*, that I could do what I really wanted to do. I don't think that I was ready for it. You know, too much freedom too fast.

He admitted that he was confused and frightened. Others saw him as being in a state that combined panic and depression. He did not look for a job or his own apartment. He rapidly assumed his former style — dressed shabbily, did not comb his hair or wash, let his room accumulate dirt, and spent his evenings watching television, saying "T.V. is my escape from myself".

That so rapid a change in role from "retarded" to "normal" was too much for John to make comfortably is hardly remarkable. Yet 9 months later he was experiencing the same problems in coping with his normal freedoms and responsibilities. During that period his work performance fluctuated but was never seen as acceptable by his supervisors. His self-esteem rose now and then, but more often fell, and his efforts to "become more normal" were unavailing. His legitimate aspirations — for a job, a car, a television set, an apartment — all failed to materialize, and not surprisingly since he refused to seek job training, or look for a job and he did not save anything from his small salary.

Instead he revelled in lurid fantasies. John admitted that his schoolmates in past years often disliked his "stories", and all who were familiar with his earlier years commented on his propensity for exaggerated and "fantasic" tales. Now he seemed to rely on his fantasies to create the normal accomplishments that in reality stayed beyond his grasp. These fantasies were presented as truth, but many could not have been since the events he reported were said to have taken place in faraway places when at the time in question, John was in his room at Vista House. His fantasies ranged from heroic athletic and sexual feats to successes in the world of business. The following verbatim examples give a sense of his state of mind when he returned to Vista after leaving for about 2 weeks early in 1974. The fabulous character of these stories is obvious. That John chose to relate these stories to an interviewer who knew a good deal about him, is also significant.[3] It is inconceivable that anyone who knew John could have believed a tale like the following, yet he told it with sincerity:

Int :   Tell me why you left (Vista House).

John: Well, I wanted to find out if I could handle being out on my own. Also, I had been in a really hairy argument with my Mom the night before.

Int :   What was that about?

John: I told her about a job that I had. I would be working in L.A. A guy would be giving me a ride to and from every day. During the weekends, I would have off. I was going to be getting paid $4.75 an hour, and I would probably be working overtime also, as a shipping clerk and just working around the shop that he had. So I called my parents to tell them, you know, I was really proud of myself being able to get this job. I had to really go out to get it. I told them that I was qualified to do it and if he didn't believe me, to try me. And he did, for a week and with no pay; I said that, "I want you to see my work". So he hired me on. I was going to start work Monday and I called her on Sunday evening and she cussed me completely out. She said things that I don't want to repeat. (She accused him of fabricating this story.) My Mom has never cussed me out in my whole life, so I hung up on her and I decided that it was time for me to split. Try to get my head together and not just let my Mom dominate me, so I took off at four o'clock in the morning.

Int :   With Carson and Donna? (friends from Vista and the workshop).

John: Right. All the way up to Las Vegas, Nevada.

Int :   Did you hitchhike?

John: Yes. After they left Las Vegas I did something that was illegal, but was a new experience for me. I got paid a little money, so I got me some nice looking clothes.

Int :   Where did you get the money?

John: From work that me and Carson were doing.

Int :   In Vegas?

John: Yes. One of the hardest places to get a job and look, we got jobs!

Int :   What kind of job?

John: Fiberglass. We were making imitation rock panels for Metro-Goldwyn-Mayer.

Int :   How did you get the job?

John: I walked into this place, I was just going in to get some water. The guy who was the contractor was there and he gave me the job like that. After Carson and Donna left I quit the job a few days after that on a Friday. I had $20.00 in my pocket so I started to boogie and I decided that I was going to get me some nice clothes and look nice and maybe I'll get me a ride east. What do I do? I go to this place. I got me an outfit dirt cheap, it was beautiful. I still have it, it's up at my best friend's place, 55 miles south of Eugene, Oregon.

Int: Where did you get the money, you only had twenty dollars?

John: I know, that's all I needed. It was at a hock shop type place and I got it dirt cheap. It fit beautifully and I got a pair of suede shoes, perfectly beautiful ones. I got a pair of pants that were crushed velvet and a matching shirt that had ruffles down the front.

Int: Just like Vegas.

John: Really. So I start boogieing down Las Vegas boulevard. Down to where I got to the strip. And so, what happens. I got five dollars left so I walked into the Sahara where this guy had lost all his money, five hundred bucks; it was gone, man. I went up to this blackjack table and I put down a dollar and if you play on scared money in Las Vegas you might as well forget it. So I said to myself I'm going to get that, I'm going to win and that's that. When I feel like I'm not going to win I'll pull it all out, cash it in and leave. Go somewhere else, maybe another table or something else, whatever turns me on at that time. I went there at ten o'clock and at midnight I stopped gambling and at that time I had five hundred dollars.

Int: You're kidding.

John: I am not kidding. So I went and bought me some more nice clothes that fit better and I went walking the strip. I saw this one hustler, a hooker. In Vegas it's illegal, also in Clark County, Reno and Lake Tahoe it's illegal prostitution. You go to a bellhop and say, "I need some entertainment, send something up". Within fifteen minutes you'll have something, whatever your specifications are. Well I got in instead of as a bell-boy, as a pimp. It was so out-of-sight, I was making all this bread, it was coming in. I was taking care of these three chicks and all of their business arrangements. I would screen them to see if they were decent dudes; I can tell pretty well. I can tell when someone is giving you a line or something. Within a week after that, each night I would come off with a thousand or five hundred bucks. And in the morning you know what would happen, I would gamble it all away.

Int: Would you lose it all?

John: You bet! I walked into Las Vegas without a cent to my name. I walked out with four hundred dollars.

Int: Did you get laid with the girls you were pimping?

John: Oh yes! There were all types of them, whatever you want they got it. For the price. If you get into the really high time, top where movie stars stay, they have chicks that go for $1,000 an hour. That's just to look at them with their clothes on, without them on it's higher. Those chicks are really high class; you can't even touch them. They are so sophisticated. My head swirled when I saw this one. Wow! The scene along that line, you can get anything you want in Vegas, if you have the money.

Int: Did you go anywhere else?

John: Really I met a lot of nice peoples, I met a lot of nasty peoples. I think the best thing that ever came about was down in Florida. I got a ride with this chick in her Mecedes Benz; she had just inherited three oil mines in Texas, a condominium in Miami Beach, Miami — one of the high class joints — and also four cocktail lounges, fancy restaurants with them. She was rolling in dough. I didn't talk about my problems, but she really digged on them. The thing that freaked me out about her was that she didn't dig on my mind. What she really dug on was my body. And that's something I never had. Her uncle had been living in Florida Everglades since he was four years old. He knew it frontwards and backwards and in between, you name it. He could take you and tell you exactly where everything was. You know how old he was? He was 79. He had been living there for 75 years. She also had scuba tanks and I love scuba diving. We went out to the Florida Keys and at the time there were not many people out there. There were maybe 5 or 10 peoples. We went way out and we were doing it in a very weird way. We didn't have clothes on; we had our tanks and that was it. It was fantastic. The water was warm, it was about 80 degrees. Can you imagine that? It was just beautiful. She also had a, you know in the Everglades they have these, I don't know what you call them . . . skin boats I guess. They have a big wheel on the back of it and they go over marshes, and water. We went on one of these.

Int: How come you left her?

John: I wanted to come back here.

Int: You're kidding.

John: That's right.

Int: You left all that for Vista House? You must have had a strong drive to come back here.

John: Like I was influenced. I really dug on this place. They helped me a lot. You heard me talking about how I couldn't stand this place. But, man, it's changed.

Int: Did things get heavy for you with the girl?

John: Oh yes, quite heavy. She wanted me to marry her, right there. I loved her, but it wouldn't be me. I would be just lazing around, I

Int: can't stand that. I'd get so bored. After we lived in the Florida
Everglades we could have gone to the Riviera and had our fun
there, and then move on from place to place, but afterwards what
would we have? Nothing, whatsoever. Then where would I be?

Int: Were you worried about your mother? Did you think about her a
lot?

John   Not very much.

Int: Have you worked that problem out pretty much?

John: Yes. If she don't like what I'm doing that's none of her business.

Int: Did you find any difference in people reacting to you differently
there than here? Because here you were called retarded for years
and you were treated like a retarded kid, right? And then you go
off on your own and nobody knows your history. Did you notice
any difference in the way people acted towards you?

John: Yes. Quite a bit of difference. They didn't put me down. I didn't
have to lie to them, I didn't have to tell them anything. I just
talked, I rapped. With this one guy it was really freaky cause
instead of me talking to him about my problems he was the one
talking to me about it. Everything he was saying to me is what I've
been telling people about the same thing. It was really freaky,
man, in him I could see what I was. I didn't put him down. I didn't
even sympathize with him. He didn't put on a sob story.

Int: What was his problem?

John: His mom had just dominated his life all his life. Very dominated.

The preposterous nature of this fabulous tale needs little comment except to
note how transparently it reveals John's feelings about his inadequacies. First,
he establishes his freedom by going to Las Vegas, that fabled place, on his
own. He then gets a job with a high salary (for 1973) without any difficulty.
Where others fail at gambling, he wins. He becomes not a mere bellboy, but a
pimp to gorgeous prostitutes. He not only has sexual relations with these
women he manages their business affairs, screens clients with a canny eye for
their acceptability and so on. His gambling achieves monumental proportions, with winnings of $1,000 each night and equivalent losses the next
morning. He then, and without explanation, finds himself in Florida where an
unbelievably wealthy heiress falls not for his mind (which he suggests would
be perfectly understandable) but for his body. She wants to marry him, but
he leaves her to return to Vista House. Somewhere in this odyssey he met a
man who talked to John about exactly the same problems John has.

Whether the information (or misinformation) he recounts came from
friends, his endless watching of television or another source, its self-aggran-
dizing character is clear. The apparent fact that he expected someone who
knew him well to accept his fantastic adventures without question is a less

improbable expectation than one might imagine. It is not uncommon for other mentally retarded persons and even direct care providers to accept just such fantastic stories. (Edgerton, 1967). Turner (1983) describes this sort of collusion, or reciprocal indulgence of one another, in a sheltered workshop society.

In the months that followed there was no perceptible change in John's life. He remained in his janitorial job at Vista House, spent most of his evenings watching T.V. in his room, and told more "success" stories. He did not look for a competitive job, save any money, or take any steps toward more independent living. The following interview illustrates John's state of mind concerning his abilities and his efforts to make the transition toward "being normal". The interview, conducted by a woman who had interviewed John as well as other residents and staff of Vista House several times before, took place in April 1974.[4]

Int: How did you feel when you were a little kid?

John: I felt inferior to other peoples, left out a lot of activities, I was Mama's boy.

Int: How old were you when you were told that you were retarded?

John: I was told when I was four.

Int: How did your Mom treat you when you were a child?

John: My Mom would keep helping me with my work, yet I thought I could do it myself, but if I did, you know, fine . . . it would be my mistake. But she wouldn't give me the chance.

Int: Did any of your playmates think of you as retarded?

John: Yes, there was one in particular.

Int: Did that bother you?

John: Yes, quite a bit because my Mom out-and-out told them that I was . . . that I was . . . that I had problems.

Int: How many years did you think of yourself as retarded?

John: Up until the age of twenty.

Int: Did you worry about other people knowing that you were retarded?

John: (with heavy sarcasm) No, I didn't need to worry. I knew my mother would tell everyone. I couldn't go out and do this and that like people did. I remember quite a few times when we went on hikes and I had to stay with her. She'd say, "Johnny, watch out, there might be a snake over there", and then all the other kids would go right on over there behind the thing where the snake was supposed to be and then she'd still tell me to "watch out", there might be a snake over there. All the other kids heard her say it.

Int: Did you believe you were limited?

John: Yes, in a lot a things. Yes (voice trails off)

Int: Which people, aside from your mother, told you that you were retarded?

John: My very best friend told me one time, "Why don't you stop trying to prove to yourself that you can do things like a normal person can do? You know that you're handicapped, that you'll never make it in school so don't try to over-work yourself."

Int: What was your reaction?

John: At the time I told him where to go and how to do it. I was thirteen at the time.

Int: Did your teachers think of you as retarded?

John: They knew I had a learning disability which was induced by my mother. Yes.

Int: Did your friends in school know you were retarded?

John: Some of 'em did. Others didn't even know. It was when I got away from my mother's apron strings that no one called me retarded, and she made sure who my friends were, they were all ones who couldn't do very much, who had something wrong with them. To where I just had to tell her, "Hey, I'm leaving". When I chose my own friends they were bad and I got in trouble for it but I learned things from it anyhow.

Int: How did you find out you weren't retarded?

John: From peoples taking tests and giving me things to do. It was three months after I started here (at Vista House).

Int: How did you feel when you found out?

John: I was astonished; I couldn't believe it. I was flabbergasted! I thought they'd made a mistake or something, so I asked 'em, "You're putting me on?" It completely went against my grain.

Int: How were things for you during the transition when you found out that you were normal?

John: It was hard, I wanted something, hey, I wanted to say, "Come here, I need some help!" And there wasn't anybody.

Int: How did your mother and father take it when they found out that you were not retarded?

John: My father took it at face value, he agreed with me. My Mom hung-up ... 'cause she had ... she didn't want to be proved wrong. It was an ego trip for her to be right. I think she's still on an ego trip.

Int: Were you considered mentally retarded at the workshop?

John: Yes, I still am. I just lived with it. I showed them I could do the work better than anyone. For a year and half's work all I had to show for it was fifty cents an hour, and that's not what I'm worth.

Int: How did you like it when you stayed in family care facilities?

John: In (the second facility) they helped me, said I could do it.

Int :   How do you like it here at Vista House?

John: I like it, I want to help people.

Int :   Do you want to move into independent living?

John: If I went into independent living right now, before I got the concept of it, of knowing about responsibility, well, I think I have to give . . . myself time to do that. I don't think I'm ready quite yet.

Int :   Why do you think you feel this way?

John: I think it's called being "institutionalized". Someone says something and they never heard it, they'd believe it. You know, if someone said sex was bad, some of these girls, they'd be wearing high collars and low skirts down to their ankles. They wouldn't let their ankles show. But if somebody told them something else they'd be altogether different.

Int :   Do any of the people here at Vista think of themselves as retarded?

John: Yes.

Int :   What does it mean to be retarded?

John: "Slow", to me it does. There's one girl that says, "I heard that there's a place where mentally retarded people go to have fun". She characterizes herself as mentally retarded. I still don't think of myself as that. You know, I won't say it.

Int :   Have you ever acted retarded?

John: A, (long pause) that's a hard question. Let's put it this way (pause). I felt like doing it but I don't think I've done it.

Int :   How does one act retarded?

John: Crazy, just . . . no . . . a rationalization: irrational, doing weird things with no cause behind it. Like running away screaming at the top of your voice. Doing things that most people would think was weird. Trying to get a lot of attention when there's no reason for it. Like that.

Int :   What did your Mom base your supposed retardation on?

John: (Making facial twitches, waving his arms and hands in spasmodic gestures, tensing his body and making a bizarre facial expression.) Acting nervous, flaky, never concentrating. Which I know I have that problem. It was supposed to be physical but I know it was psychological. I've calmed myself quite a bit.

Int :   What problems did you have making the transition from being retarded to being a normal person?

John: I tried to act more mature which was very hard. Still is very hard. I hadn't really grown-up. I was below most people in maturity.

Int :   Is it easier to be retarded?

John: Yeah, you better believe it. You're sheltered you know, you don't have to take on the responsibility of an adult and everyone, I think, wants to be sheltered. I mean, once in awhile. Once in a month I just want to . . . when I have problems I can't cope with I say, "John, let's go back where I was and act like a little kid again".

Int: What has been your biggest problem since you learned you weren't retarded?

John: Being on my own. I don't think I can handle it.

Int: Did you ever think before about what it would be like to be not retarded, before they told you you weren't retarded?

John: No.

Int: You just accept it?

John: Yeah, simple, I could take it.

Int: Do you find it makes a difference in how people think of you?

John: Yeah, some people, they put me on a pedestal and say, "Hey, he's retarded, leave him alone, don't bother him". When they don't know that I'm retarded, they act like I know how to cope with life. Makes me feel good but other times it freaks me completely out. I think, "How am I supposed to act now?" If I flub up now I may as well hang it up for good.

Int: How do some of the people here, retarded people, feel about going back to the institution (a large state hospital) they come from?

John: Everyone hates the institution, they don't ever want to go back. Some of them, like Georgia, she don't want to go back. They treated her real mean there. They locked her in a small room gave shock therapy and all kinds of other things.

Int: How do you feel about the workshop?

John: Oh, the workshop, I mean, these training centers are a bunch of bullhonky because they never have normal peoples work on the same level as these people. It's a shame to alienate them that way. I think they should put them on a real job and tell them, "you're going to ack like a real adult". They tell them that, then they treat them like children. They tell them, "You're an adult, you're 'young adults'" (now getting very agitated) but then they treat them like children. If you (interviewer) didn't clean up your driveway at home, you know, you're in an independent living situation, but if you didn't clean your driveway at home, you wouldn't be put on restriction like they do here. That's plain silly. What you should do is show them the real world. Make them learn what it's like in the community, that it's not all peaches and cream. Uhm, uhm, a lot of these kids, I call them kids because they are, they don't take on responsibility.

Int: How do you feel about the family care homes you were in?

John: A bunch of bullhonky.

Int: Why?

John: Because the people that run them don't know what they're doing. They just run them for the money, not to help people. All you do in those places is sleep, eat, go to the bathroom, go to the work-shop and watch TV. Every so often a little recreation here and there. And then they let everyone else around the block know there are M. R.'s in there and tell them to stay away from them. They aren't given any type of freedom. There's always someone to keep an eye on them. (At this point John's supervisor at Vista House walks up to the interviewer and asks, "Is it okay if he leaves for a minute?" Interviewer agrees).

Supervisor to John: "You got a certain amount of work to do here and that there kitchen still looks like hell."

John: (voice quivering) "I've been working on it, I've got it three-quarters done."

Supervisor: (angrily) "It's supposed to be done by 11:30 and I don't think it's ever been done by then".

John: (looking as if he's about to cry) Yes it has!

Supervisor: "I got on you once today, how many times I got to do it." (At this point without another word the supervisor walks away. John sits head down, picking at the grass, looking as if there are tears in his eyes).

Int :   (tentatively) . . . How does that makes you feel?

John: (Looking up slowly and struggling to control his voice) I take it . . . I don't let it make me feel . . . because I know he doesn't know what he's talking about.

Int :   Why do you think he does it?

John: Because he don't take on that responsibility. He's worse than I am (his voice recovering now). Oh, I know I'm lazy, but he is, well, what you call a male chauvinist pig, if you want to know the truth. I put him down more times than anyone and he's never come up with an answer. He only wanted to put me down in front of you.

Int :   How do you feel about working here?

John: Oh, I want to work here as a counselor and help peoples. Not as a janitor, that's . . . I think really, I have more potential than that. I want to help peoples. That would be a real thrill.

Int :   What do you think is hardest for you, to accept the fact that you're not retarded or for others who knew you as retarded to accept the fact that you're not retarded?

John: For people who thought of me as retarded.

Nothing changed significantly in John's life for 3 months after this interview. At that point, John suddenly left Vista House, purportedly to stay with a friend in rural Oregon. We were unable to learn anything reliable about his life since that time. While it would certainly have been desirable to observe

John's post-delabeling adaptation for longer than the year available to us, some important conclusion nevertheless seem warranted.

John was delabeled from the status of a mentally retarded person, to that of a person of average intelligence. The expectations of those persons most responsible for his future were consistent with his new status; with the sole exception of his mother, he was expected to make a rapid transition to independent living, self-support and social competence. Six months was considered ample time for him to achieve these goals. One year later he had achieved none of them. Seventeen years of socialization for incompetence were not to be erased by "closing a file".

SOCIALIZATION FOR INCOMPETENCE

The complex of expectations and practices that produces socialization for incompetence begins with the imposition of restrictions that deny mentally retarded children access to experiences that are commonplace for other, non-retarded children. For the retarded child, certain experiences are too dangerous or too difficult. Not all parents restrict experience in these ways, and not many are as extreme as John's adoptive mother, but nevertheless, most parents *do* deny their mentally retarded children experiences that they would allow for, or encourage, in their "normal" children. Subtle joking, teasing and instructive interchanges based on nuances of language and shared knowledge are replaced by direct didactic or corrective strategies, often calling for the parent to intervene and complete problematic behavior for the retarded child. More overt restrictions include efforts to avoid risk and limit responsibility in such matters as physical aggression, sports, bicycle riding, choice of playmates or simply the use of tools, kitchen knives or the need to care for household pets.

The experience of adolescents and young adults must be even more circumscribed than those for children. Now, sexuality must be restricted along with smoking, drinking or operating motor vehicles. Koegel's previous example in this volume should serve. When the retarded son of a well-educated and affluent set of parents first expressed an interest in alcohol, he was encouraged to drink as much as he possibly could so that the resulting extreme nausea and hangover would teach him never to drink again. It did. When his non-retarded brother expressed a similar interest, his drinking was closely instructed and supervised by his father so that he could learn how much alcohol he could soberly tolerate.

These kinds of restrictions, arguably reasonable for some more severely incompetent, mentally retarded children, nevertheless additively reduce social competence. As Koegel reported in an earlier chapter, a child who had been told not to touch sharp knives all his life can easily, as a young man in our sample did, prove to be unable to use a sharp kitchen knife for a simple task at the age of 25. Some parents come to understand how their restrictions

may have been unwise especially as their children become adults. As
Kaufman said in her paper in this volume, referring to her past restrictions of
her retarded daughter Colette's behavior and freedom, and the conflicts that
ensued: "Now I wonder if it may not be too harsh a regimen. There are many
kinds of success: the one that is most meaningful for her may turn out to be
centered around all-night sessions with friends, a baby or two, and SSI for
income. Ten months ago I would have shuddered at that scenario. Today I
would be a good deal more accepting if it occurred."

When mildly retarded young adults leave their parents' homes to live in
"group homes", their access to normal experience continues to be restricted.
Certain behaviors are still seen as too dangerous or difficult, but in addition
to these reasons for restrictions, group home caretakers are usually under
great pressure to manage and control several "residents" with limited time,
energy and money. The result has been described before (Edgerton, 1975;
Bercovici, 1980). The retarded person is isolated from non-retarded persons
and from ordinary experience. Residents are typically compelled to eat
together, work together and even have "recreation" together. As Bercovici
has put it, they are "herded" with few opportunities to plan, make decisions,
take risks or make mistakes. Even time is planned and structured for them.
Moreover, it is common for residents to be denied access to such every day
experiences as using a telephone, doing household chores, using money,
making friends or planning for tomorrow. Sheltered workshops sometimes
provide greater autonomy or teach useful skills, but workshops too impose
restrictions on normal experiences (Turner, 1983).

Compliance with the regimentation and restricted autonomy of community
residential and vocational settings is sometimes brought about by the use of
subtle psychological practices such as the use of terms like "Mom" and "Kid"
to place care-taker and resident in a familiar parent-child role of authority
and dependency. More coercive tactics are also employed. The rebellious
resident or worker may be subjected to subtle or non-so-subtle threats such
as transfer to a large state hospital, loss of a desired job or friend, or termina-
tion of "benefits" such as S.S.I. Mentally retarded persons are easily cowed by
threats such as these since they regularly overestimate the power and legal
authority of caretakers to control their lives. When these means of assuring
compliance fail, caretakers employ others. Residents are often over-medi-
cated with neuroleptic drugs and are sometimes abused physically. For
example they are commonly "restricted" to their rooms. When, as is usually
the case, there is no one in the "outside" world to whom the retarded person
can appeal, compliance is the only alternative. Their world of experience
remains restricted.

As much as it is in the interest of group home caretakers not to encourage
more independent behavior lest economic loss be incurred when a resident
leaves and is not replaced by another (a commonly expressed fear on the
part of caretakers), it is also in the interest of many residents to accept their

restricted lives without too much complaint. The regulations concerning receipt of S.S.I. provide bureaucratic support for this pattern (Estroff, 1981). The experience of John illustrate the fact that there are benefits to be had in accepting dependency and restriction as a way of life. There is no need to rise early each day, cope with the demands of the work-place, solve practical problems of money management, bill-paying, and the like. One need not save for tomorrow, groom oneself well, plan ahead and defer to the needs and requirements of strangers in a complex and competitive world. A set routine, few demands, television, and one's fantasy, can, after all, amount to a pleasant way of life, at least when the alternatives are so unpleasant.

SOME PRACTICAL AND THEORETICAL IMPLICATIONS OF DELABELING

Substantial numbers of persons who have been eligible for services due to mental retardation are losing that eligibility — and the label with it — when they are found to have I.Q.'s well above 70. If eligibility standards become more stringent, even larger numbers may be delabeled. Agency personnel have often expected delabeled persons to become more normal in short order; if our research is correct, assumption of a more normal role will be slow and agonizing, if indeed, it happens at all. Failure to recognize the difficulties such people face will only impose upon them an insupportable burden.

If our interpretation of the data before us is correct, then it is also necessary to suggest a cautionary note for those in the field of mental retardation who continue to refer to the effects of labeling as if that "act" had impressive, even ineluctable, life consequences. In present-day reality, the label is seldom imposed in such a way that it has cataclysmic effects on its recipient; instead, labels are poorly defined, poorly understood, and may be more or less known to the mentally retarded person. Their more direct effect is on parents, teachers and providers of services in the mental retardation system. Once labeled persons enter this world, they are vulnerable to the expectations and practices we have discussed, and when they are exposed to such socialization experiences in a concerted way, they take on incompetent and dependent roles.

It is the sub-culture within which persons are socialized that determines their competence, not the event of labeling. This is, of course, perfectly consistent with "labeling" or "societal reaction" theory, but is too seldom taken fully to heart by those who attempt to care for, or theorize about, mentally retarded persons.

NOTES

1. I gratefully acknowledge support for this research from NICHD Grant No. HD 04612, the

Mental Retardation Research Center, UCLA, and NICHD Program Project Grant No. HD 11944—02, The Community Adaptation of Mildly Retarded Persons. I am also grateful to Sylvia Bercovici and Judith R. Myers for their contributions in collecting much of the material presented here.
2. This estimate is based on the estimates of 2 Regional Center directors in the Los Angeles area. It is an estimate but an informed one.
3. The interviewer, Judith R. Myers, was familiar with many aspects of John's life as he knew.
4. This interview was video-taped by Judith R. Myers.

REFERENCES

Becker, H. S.
   1963 *Outsiders: Studies in the sociology of deviance.* New York: Free Press.
Bercovici, S. M.
   1981 The deinstitutionalization of the mentally retarded persons: Ethnographic research in community environments. *In* R. H. Bruininks, C. E. Meyers, B. B. Sigford and K. C. Lakin (eds.), *Deinstitutionalization and community adjustment of mentally retarded people* (pp. 133—144) (Monograph No. 4). Washington D.C.: American Association on Mental Deficiency.
Deacon, J. J.
   1974 *Joey.* New York: Charles Scribner's Sons.
Dexter, L. A.
   1956 Towards a sociology of the mentally defective. *American Journal of Mental Deficiency, 61*: 10—16.
Dexter, L. A.
   1958 A social theory of mental deficiency. *American Journal of Mental Deficiency, 62*: 920—928.
Dusek, J. B.
   1975 Do teachers bias children's learning? *Review of Educational Research, 45*: 661—684.
Edgerton, R. B.
   1967 The cloak of competence: Stigma in the lives of the mentally retarded. Berkeley and Los Angeles: University of California Press.
Edgerton, R. B.
   1975 Issues relating to the quality of life among mentally retarded persons. *In* M. Begab and S. Richardson (eds.), *The mentally retarded and society: A social science perspective* (pp. 127—140). Baltimore: University Park Press.
Edgerton, R. B. and Langness, L. L.
   1978 Observing mentally retarded persons in community settings: An anthropological perspective. *In* G. P. Sackett (ed.), *Observing behavior Vol. I: Theory and applications in mental retardation* (pp. 335—348). Baltimore: University Park Press.
Estroff, S. E.
   1981 *Making it crazy: An ethnography of psychiatric clients in an American community.* Berkeley: University of California Press.
Goffman, E.
   1961 *Asylums: Essays on the social situations of mental patients and other inmates.* New York: Anchor Books.
Guskin, S. L.
   1978 Theoretical and empirical strategies for the study of the labeling of mentally retarded persons. *In* N. R. Ellis (ed.), *International Review of Research in Mental Retardation, Vol. 9* (pp. 127—158). New York: Academic Press.

Hobbs, N. (ed.)
   1975   *Issues in the classification of children.* (Vols. 1 and 2). San Francisco: Jossey-Bass.
Klemke, L. W. and Tiedeman, G. H.
   1981   Toward an understanding of false accusation: The pure case of deviant labeling. *Deviant Behavior, 2*: 261—285.
Lemert, E. M.
   1951   *Social pathology.* New York: McGraw-Hill.
MacMillan, D. L.
   1977   *Mental retardation in school and society.* Boston: Little, Brown and Son.
MacMillan, D. L., Jones, R. L. and Aloia, G. F.
   1974   The mentally retarded label: a theoretical analysis and review of research. *American Journal of Mental Deficiency, 79*: 241—261.
McQueen, R.
   1970   Larry: Case history of a mistake. *In* B. Blatt (ed.), *Souls in extremis: An anthology of victims and victimizers* (pp. 199—208). Boston: Allyn and Bacon.
Mercer, J.
   1973   *Labeling the retarded.* Berkeley: University of California Press.
Mercer, J. R.
   1970   Sociology perspectives on mild mental retardation. *In* H. C. Haywood (ed.), *Socio-cultural aspects of mental retardation.* New York: Appleton-Century Crofts.
Rosenthal, R. and Jacobson, L.
   1968   *Pygmalion in the classroom: Teacher expectation and pupils' intellectual development.* New York: Holt, Rinehart and Winston.
Rowitz, L.
   1981   A sociological perspective on labeling in mental retardation. *Mental Retardation, 19*: 47—51.
Sagarin, E.
   1975   *Deviants and deviance.* New York: Praeger.
Scott, R. A.
   1969   *The making of blind men.* New York: Russell Sage.
Tannenbaum, F.
   1938   *Crime and the community.* Boston: Gunn.
Turner, J. L.
   1980   Yes I am human: Autobiography of a "retarded career". *Journal of Community Psychology, 8*: 3—8.
Turner, J. L.
   1983   Workshop society: Ethnographic observations in a work setting for retarded adults. *In* K. Kernan, M. Begab and R. Edgerton (eds.), *Environments and behavior: The adaption of mentally retarded persons* (pp. 147—171). Baltimore: University Park Press.
Yoshida, R.
   1974   *Effects of labeling on elementary and EMR teacher's expectancies for change in a student's performance.* Unpublished doctoral dissertation, University of Southern California.
Zigler, E. and Balla, D.
   1977   Impact of institutional experience on the behavior and development of retarded persons. *American Journal of Mental Deficiency, 82*: 1—11.

PAUL KOEGEL

SOCIAL SUPPORT AND INDIVIDUAL ADAPTATION:
A DIACHRONIC PERSPECTIVE

Over the last ten years, increasing attention has been focused on a phenomenon referred to as "social support". The helping professions, and even
the community-at-large, bear witness to the growing popularity of this term:
the phrases "social support" and "support systems" have quickly found their
place in the general lexicon, being used regularly to refer to the social
resources available to an individual both on a day-to-day basis and during
times of crisis. One could just as readily look toward the scientific community for confirmation of the excitement which these concepts have
generated: researchers from many disciplines have looked toward social
support and support systems as variables to be scrutinized for their potential
effect on any number of outcomes pertaining to the larger question of
individual adaptation.

   Although consistent use of the term social support is relatively new, the
concept can hardly be heralded as a recent one. All efforts to understand the
behavior of people-in-society have implicitly shared the assumption that the
successful adaptation of individuals rests heavily on the nature of their ties to
other individuals and social institutions. In cultural anthropology alone,
countless ethnographers have depicted how kin, economic, political, religious, and other cultural institutions create webs of reciprocal social obliga-
tions which serve, among other things, to meet individual needs. Urban
anthropologists have described how migrants to urban centers depend on
such ties for material assistance, emotional support, and the information
needed to successfully adjust to a strange setting and a new way of life
(Basham, 1978; Gulick, 1974; Snyder, 1976). Medical anthropologists have
realized that disturbances in social relationships may profoundly affect
individual physical and psychological equilibrium, and have documented how
treatment often involves the attempt to mend disrupted social ties (Clark,
1970; Fox, 1964; Freed and Freed, 1964; Turner, 1964) or to create new
ones (Crapanzano, 1973; Kennedy, 1967; Lewis, 1966). Indeed, a great deal
of anthropology and the social sciences in general can be seen as touching on
the question of social support.

   Recent applications of the term social support differ from these more
general and implicit usages in that they involve the attempt to define and
operationalize social support as a variable and to apply it to the investigation
of a specific set of problems through the use of quantitative techniques.
These efforts have not been without serious flaws (Koegel, 1982), but they
have yielded a growing understanding of the important role which social
support plays in enabling people to maintain their health and to meet the

127

L. L. Langness and H. G. Levine (eds.), Culture and Retardation, 127–153.
© 1986 by D. Reidel Publishing Company.

vicissitudes of life. A voluminous literature now attests to the way in which the instrumental and emotional resources available to individuals affect their ability to cope with stressful events, whether they be pregnancy (Nuckolls *et al.*, 1972), myocardial infarction (Finlayson, 1976), unemployment (Gore, 1978), or bereavement (Walker *et al.*, 1977). (For reviews of this literature see Cassell, 1974, 1975; Cobb, 1976; Dean and Lin, 1977; Kaplan, Cassell and Gore, 1977; Pilisuk and Froland, 1978.) Examinations of the social support systems of normal as opposed to neurotic, psychotic, and schizophrenic individuals have suggested that psychologically impaired individuals do not have the same access to support resources as do individuals showing no psychological symptoms (Cohen and Sokolovsky, 1978; Garrison, 1978; Hammer *et al.*, 1978; Froland *et al.*, 1979; Henderson, 1977; Lin *et al.*, 1973; Pattison *et al.*, 1975; Pilisuk and Froland, 1978; Winefield, 1979). Likewise, research with the elderly has pointed to the important relationship between social support and health as well as quality of life (Lowenthal and Haven, 1968; Lopata, 1975; Maxwell, 1979; Gelein, 1980; Wan, 1982).

While it is true that these efforts have contributed significantly to an appreciation of how support systems function to enable individuals to meet particular sets of environmental demands, it is also true that they have been restricted to single points in time. One consequence of this, unintended though it may be, is that support systems are treated as though they were fixed and unchanging entities, remaining stable over time. Admittedly this is in part an unavoidable artifact of the process of counting and measuring, for to do so one must freeze the phenomenon at hand. But the fact remains that change is an inevitable aspect of social relationships, and that support systems are thus often in flux. Relatively short periods of time may find them undergoing minor and even major changes, and long periods of time will undoubtedly see the occurrence of radical shifts in individual support resources (Koegel, 1982).

If the larger theoretical purpose of studying support systems lies in examining their impact on individual adaptation — a concept which by definition implies continuing change and adjustment over time — a more processual and longitudinal approach would seem to be a necessary complement to the synchronic approaches employed thus far. An approach which incorporates a diachronic perspective would allow examination of the way in which individual needs, circumstances, and support systems constantly change over time, and how changes in each affect the other. In focusing attention on how changes in support systems affect, and are affected by, circumstances and needs over the course of individual lives, such an approach would ultimately lay the groundwork for a dynamic appreciation of the relationship between social support and individual adaptation.

The life history method would appear to be one logical means of exploring how support systems change over time and the consequences of such change for individual adaptation. A life history, constructed from the combined perspectives offered by an individual, by others involved with the individual, by direct observation, and by any number of supplemental sources (Langness, 1965; Langness and Frank, 1981), can provide rich data on both the shifting resources available to a person as his or her social network is modified and the resulting changes in an individual's life circumstances. Moreover, because life histories focus not only on actors and events but on personality, self-defined needs, coping styles, and the way in which an individual subjectively perceives his or her experiences, a life history can also contribute to an understanding of how factors unique to the individual feed into the relationships between changing support systems and individual adaptation.

By way of example, this chapter presents an abbreviated life history of a woman whose many and varied experiences are as intrinsically interesting as they are revealing of issues pertaining to the study of social support. Penny Davis was one of 40 adults who formed the research sample of a project aimed at exploring the impact of social support on the attempts of mildly retarded individuals to live independently of parents and caretakers, and on the general quality of their lives. Research with this sample was conducted from September 1980 to December 1981 though many of these individuals, Penny included, had participated in previous research projects as well. The multi-method approach employed included structured interviews and more intensive qualitative techniques, all of which took place against the backdrop provided by ongoing participant-observation. In addition, basic life history information was collected on each of these research participants, and more detailed life histories on a smaller number of individuals. A closer look at one of these life histories reveals the very crucial role which support systems play in the lives of the mildly retarded. But even more, it reveals the dramatic changes that support systems can undergo over time, the implications of these changes for an individual's life style, and the importance of attending to an individual's own perception of her existence.

PENNY DAVIS DESCRIBED

Although Penny Davis would never be described as a beauty, she is certainly a pleasant looking woman who appears somewhat older than her 39 years, a result, perhaps, of being somewhat portly, though by no means obese. Her blue eyes, freckles, ruddy complexion, and engaging smile are framed by short, curly hair; together with her large frame, these features somehow call to mind a sturdy Irish matron. Her rather casual attitude toward cleanliness, grooming, and general self-presentation do little to enhance her looks — her hair is more often than not matted with grease; her incongruous outfits (a dress, for instance, worn over a t-shirt such that the shirt protrudes at the neck and sleeves) are customarily stained and soiled; her body commonly emits a noticeable odor born of an aversion of bathing.

But Penny's most striking characteristics have much less to do with her looks than they do her personality. An incredibly gregarious woman, Penny readily and aggressively engages in social interaction with anyone who will respond to her overtures. At McDonald's, she inserts her opinions into a private discussion between a group of men regarding the phone company. On the street, she stops to chat with a couple about their dog and eventually nudges the conversation in other directions. In a parking lot, she expresses interest in a man's camper. Often she is ignored or rebuffed. Equally often she is tolerated and even encouraged. As a result, her network of acquaintances reaches far and wide, and while she often has trouble remembering the names of these new "buddies", her memory is infallible when it comes to their occupations, family relationships, illnesses, and other critical incidents in their lives.

In many ways, Penny seems to fit one long-term stereotype of the mildly retarded woman: innocent, trusting, devoid of the perceptiveness and savvy she needs to protect herself, and above all, promiscuous. She is hardly discriminating in both the overtures she makes and accepts. She blithely enters the cars of men she has met only minutes before, with no thought of her personal safety. She confidently invites men with questionable motives and of equally questionable appearance into her house for a beer or even to spend the night, with little consideration of the potential consequences. She is easily convinced by a new boyfriend to sell a valuable possession in order to raise money to repair his car. She is ready at the drop of a hat to accept the invitation of a relative stranger to leave Los Angeles and accompany him virtually anywhere.

But to say that Penny has difficulty in rejecting the advances of men is not to say that she is completely guileless or equally malleable in all situations. While she can easily be talked into potentially dangerous situations or out of valuable possessions, she can, when an issue is important to her, stubbornly hold her ground. Further, she is capable of being manipulative in her attempts to get others to carry out her wishes, and is not above losing her temper and exploding if pushed too far. She exercises a significant amount of control over conversations in both intentional and unintentional ways, changing topics frequently, long before her conversational partner feels the current one has been exhausted, and visibly withdrawing when the subject is one which she feels is unpleasant.

Penny's conversational style, in fact, has been the bane of the existence of the three field researchers by whom she has been visited over the course of the last five and a half years. While more than willing to have a field researcher tag along with her or take her out for lunch, Penny is by no means introspective and actively dodges questions aimed at eliciting her feelings about, and memories of, times past. Caught in a rare receptive mood, she can be informative and expansive; caught in an uncooperative frame of mind, she can tie a field researcher into knots by contradicting herself, by dropping bits of information but rapidly changing the subject, or by simply stonewalling certain avenues of inquiry.

Over the course of research contact, however, a rather comprehensive picture of Penny's life has emerged through a variety of sources. Penny was first contacted by a field researcher in July, 1976. With the exception of two nine month periods of time, she was visited regularly by field researchers through December, 1981. During certain periods, visits took place as frequently as once a week with additional phone contact; at other times, they occurred as infrequently as every six weeks. Field visits included a blend of conversation on a wide range of topics and observation of Penny in her habitual haunts, both alone and with her friends and acquaintances. Interviews were also conducted with as many individuals in her life as were willing to lend their perspective — her paternal aunt, a close friend, a social worker, a Regional Center counselor, boyfriends, her cousin, occupational therapists, neighbors, and so forth. The combination of what Penny and all of these people said about her past and present, as well as our own observations of the myriad happenings in her life during the time we have known her, reveal a fascinating portrait of a life in process and a changing support system over time.

AN OVERVIEW OF PENNY'S LIFE

Penny was born in 1942 in a Salvation Army home for unwed mothers. Her biological mother, who was 13 at the time, immediately, even if reluctantly, gave her up for adoption to a great-aunt and uncle (Olivia and Bob Davis) who had no other children. It came as quite a surprise to the friends and neighbors of this couple when they announced that they were adopting a child. Most agreed that Olivia in particular had never expressed interest in children and did not really seem prepared to assume the responsibilities of motherhood. A number of individuals attributed this sudden move to the birth of Olivia's niece and her jealousy over the attention showered on her sister and her baby. Olivia, they speculated, was anxious to adopt this child so that she too could have a child as perfect as Laura.

Sadly, Penny, according to relatives and life-long neighbors, quickly showed signs that she would not be the perfect child her mother had envisioned. Said one neighbor,

Olivia and Bob never should have taken her. People tried to tell them there was something wrong with her, even when she was a tiny little thing. By the time Penny was six months old, anyone could see that she wasn't normal. And by the time she was a year old it was clearly evident. She just wasn't doing the things a year old baby could do. I don't think the child walked until she was two and a half. And I don't think she spoke a word until she was close to three. So you see, she had a very bad start.

Olivia, however, refused to believe that there was anything wrong and insisted to anyone that suggested otherwise that Penny was perfectly allright. She was forced to face the fact that Penny had certain problems when, at age three, she had her first seizure (*petit mal*). But she adamantly denied that Penny might be retarded even as the evidence mounted, dismissing any aberrant behavior noted by neighbors, who compared her to the other young children on the street, as a temporary result of the seizures. "And even after she started school", reported the neighbor, "if the teacher sent home notes saying that the child needed special attention or tutoring, Olivia would just cuss out the teachers and say they didn't know what they were talking about".

As much as people worried over both Olivia's parenting skills and her emotional capacity for mothering, they generally acknowledged that Penny was a well-loved child who wanted for little as she was growing up — if anything, she was pampered and spoiled. Her primary ties were in the neighborhood, where everyone felt sorry for her and tried to be kind, and where she played with younger children, having been shunned by her peers. Even her social contact with the younger children was restricted at times when mothers refused to allow their children to play with her, noting that her caring, affectionate behavior could quickly and radically shift to meanness. Penny may very well have learned of such behavior shifts at home. Olivia, according to many accounts, grew increasingly disenchanted as the years passed. She loved Penny, but could be kind one moment, ignore Penny the next, and then just as quickly demand that she complete chores which had never been her responsibility, threatening to beat her with a coat hanger if she failed to do so. Penny's paternal aunt somewhat shamefully admitted that Olivia was known to lock Penny in a closet in the back bedroom and beat her on many occasions. Penny's father, who was devoted to her, did his best to intervene but he too was said to be afraid of his wife and relatively ineffectual in the face of her anger. Penny herself, who only rarely talked about her parents ("They're dead. I don't like to talk about them too much. It makes me upset when I talk about them.") remembered her father's efforts to stand up for her and commented on them more than once. Asked if she liked one parent more than the other on one occasion, she confessed, "Half the time it was my father because when my mother'd try to hit me, he'd stand up for me."

Little is remembered about Penny's school years and even the question of whether or not she was formally labeled at that point remains unclear. It is clear, however, that while Penny had been pushed through the previous grades in spite of her poor math skills and low level of proficiency in writing, high school proved to be more of a problem. Penny attended her first year only intermittently and dropped out shortly thereafter. Meanwhile, Olivia, whose drinking through the years had gotten progressively out of hand, had truly become an alcoholic. Having taught Penny early on how to use the bus system, it was now easy to give her money and send her off to wherever she wanted to go. Penny's life thus settled into a new routine. She would leave for work in the morning with her father, who "employed" her at his bicycle shop, arriving there at 7:30 a.m. She would carry out her duties — sweeping and dusting — but would soon be out on the street in front of the store, chatting with passersby. By 10:30 she would take off and begin a daily routine of wandering, taking the bus to the beach, a pier, a mall, or any number of spots which became regular haunts. Her father placed few restrictions on her; her mother only erratically applied discipline. Thus Penny was relatively independent and learned to cherish her autonomy. More and more, she involved herself with buddies and boyfriends encountered on her daily jaunts.

Penny's life changed little when Olivia died in 1972 of cancer of the liver. Olivia had been sick for a while and the family, including Penny, was aware for some time that the illness was terminal. Penny gave no outward signs of grieving at her mother's death, unlike her reaction in June of 1975 when her father, at age 67, had a heart attack on a Sunday night while at home and died the next day — Penny, who was at the shop on that Monday morning, became hysterical with grief. Life did change for Penny at this point. At the age of 33, with her last adopted parent gone and her biological mother (who was married with four children) refusing to take any responsibility for her, Penny was alone. Her father had consistently refused to face the reality that he would die, and had brushed off relatives when they pressed him on what would become of Penny. But he did leave a will bequeathing the house and the remainder of his estate to Penny, placed in a trust to be administered by Laura and her parents. No provisions were made, however, for anyone to assume responsibility for overseeing the day-to-day aspects of Penny's life.

The attitude of Penny's relatives, who resented the responsibility which had been foisted on them, was initially one of *laissez-faire*. Uncle Burt, Aunt Marjorie and Laura, the trustees, lived in Pasadena, and were content to have as little actual contact with Penny as they could manage. They perceived their role to be to manage Penny's financial affairs, not her life. An arrangement was worked out whereby they sent a weekly allowance to Mrs. Pelham, an aunt who had always lived down the street from Penny, and she doled the money out in three installments over the course of the week. Mrs. Pelham saw Penny regularly and reported back to the Davises when she felt Penny was in need of clothes or anything else that would require a larger expenditure. But she too avoided interfering in Penny's life as much as possible, both because of a natural reluctance to confront the headstrong woman and because of her own preoccupation with her husband's progressive senility.

Penny thus found herself with even more freedom than before. While her standards of domestic activity fell dramatically short of those of her aunts and neighbors, she was content with the way she was running her life. With the money she received from the trust she would shop for groceries, cooking for herself when the spirit moved her, eating out frequently, and doting on her cat and dog. Slowly the house absorbed the odor of kitty litter, dirty dog, and unwashed clothes, as did Penny, but this did not bother her. Her days continued to be filled with expeditions to local hang-outs — gas stations, fire stations, donut shops, coffee shops — where she continued to meet friends, mostly men. However, she could now bring them home, and she did. A parade of men, the majority of whom sent shivers up the spine of Mrs. Pelham, passed through the house within the first six months of her father's death. Two of these men, in fact, lived there for a couple of months, helping themselves to Penny's possessions and sharing her allowance.

While Penny's relatives turned their heads and ignored what they saw as Penny's unbecoming and unconventional behavior, they felt compelled to become involved when they realized, in January of 1976, that Penny was close to five months pregnant. Penny was excited about the upcoming birth and convinced that the father, who was living with her, would marry her. Aunt Marjorie and Uncle Burt, however, pressured Penny into both an abortion and a tubal ligation. Shortly thereafter, Penny's boyfriend disappeared. Penny remains bitter over this turn of events, and only occasionally acknowledges her inability to bear a child. As much as a year after the abortion, she wistfully commented,

I used to cry and miss him, else I would had him right now. The baby's name would have been Jonathan. He'd a been six months old. This was David Jonathan's baby, the one that was supposed to marry me. He came home one day and says, "I thought you were going to have a baby". And I says, "Yeah, my s.o.b aunt and uncle made me have an abortion". And he says, "Aren't we gonna have the baby?". And I says, "No, they made me give it up". He was so upset about it and that was when he left me . . .

Whereas up to that point the relatives had been content to allow Penny to live life as she chose, her pregnancy led them to scrutinize her life style and to re-evaluate their *laissez-faire* policy. They found it increasingly difficult to ignore Penny's promiscuity. They eyed with concern Penny's habit of bundling her beloved animals into a baby stroller, covering them snugly with a blanket and wheeling them around the neighborhood for their evening constitutional, and were convinced that she was a laughing stock. Moreover, they were troubled by the deteriorating condition of Penny's trust, probate having taken much of what had originally been a substantial amount. The solution, they decided, was to sell the house and place Penny in a board and care facility. Upon making the decision, Uncle Burt contacted the Regional Center for the Developmentally Disabled,[1] which in turn referred him to the Continuing Care Services Section (CCSS) of what was then the State Department of Health — CCSS was responsible at that time for all out-of-home placements.[2] In July, 1976, the case was assigned to Eloise Barnard, a social worker.

Eloise Barnard viewed the idea of a move to a board and care with skepticism, concerned that the relatives were forcing Penny into a restrictive and inappropriate environment simply to end their unwanted responsibility for her actions. Speaking directly with Penny, she learned that Penny was reluctant to either move from the neighborhood, which she knew so well, give up her animals, or sacrifice her freedom of movement. While recognizing the relatives' concern over Penny's life style, she dismissed their preoccupation with the neighbors' opinions, citing that most had known Penny all of her life. She also insisted that taking away Penny's animals would be unwise following the coerced abortion. She decided that Penny needed a "socialization" program. Once that was accomplished, she could live in her own apartment, thus allowing the house to be sold.

Having convinced the Davises to allow an occupational therapist to see Penny regularly in order to teach her household skills, and having decided to enroll Penny in a living skills class at her local high school's night school, Mrs. Barnard set out to inform Penny of these new developments. Stopping off at Mrs. Pelham's house, she learned that Penny had been entertaining a phone company serviceman who had just left. Asked if he was a boyfriend, Penny replied that he was just a "buddy". Mrs. Barnard felt this was a good time to "bring up the subject of heterosexual relations" and lectured Penny on the need to be more discriminating in her behavior. She then informed Penny of the plans for the occupational therapist and night school. Penny's reaction was one of anger, tears, and resentment. She did not want a relative stranger coming into her house telling her what to do.

Nevertheless, Mrs. Barnard set up a meeting to introduce Penny to the therapist. At that meeting, set at Penny's home (which she had more than adequately cleaned for the occasion), Mrs. Barnard explained that "the purpose in bringing Bonnie here and going to class tonight is to help you learn to take care of yourself. Otherwise, in the board and care home, you won't have freedom." From there, the conversation moved to meal plans, a balanced diet, the virtues of cleanliness, the need for regular trips to the laundromat, budgeting and record keeping, and so forth. Bonnie, it was decided, would visit twice a week.

While Penny tacitly went along with Mrs. Barnard's plans, her feelings ran counter to them. Night school, in her mind, was an unwanted infringement, interfering with the schedules of some of her working men friends who dropped by in the evenings. And Bonnie, she felt, was a busybody who had no business telling a 34 year old woman how to run her life. Bonnie's prescriptions for life were not Penny's. Penny was not unaware of how to do certain tasks, or of the availability of certain food items — she simply wanted to do things her own way according to her own timetable. She thus endured Bonnie's visits but refused to follow her advice once she was gone. At one point, full of resentment at Bonnie's intervention, she offered,

Bonnie was saying that she's here to help me cook. I can do my own cooking. I don't need her to help me cook. She gets me so damn mad half the time. I feel like telling her off. That day we went to the store she made me use that whole eleven dollars and I only got two dollars back. You should have seen all the stuff I didn't want to get. I didn't want to get any corn — she made me get that. I didn't want to get any apples or bananas right now — she made me get that. I didn't want to get any lettuce or tomatoes right now — she made me get that. I wanted to get some meat and some small stuff. You should see the refrigerator right now — It's unbelievable. And we ended up going to the market at 3:00 on Friday afternoon. That's ridiculous — you wouldn't believe how crowded it was. I usually go on Wednesday mornings — it's much less crowded then.

Penny found many ways to hinder Bonnie's agenda. Resenting Bonnie's tendency to tell her what to cook or bake, she made sure that she had prepared something to her liking before Bonnie arrived. Displeased with Bonnie's insistence that she buy certain items, she allowed them to spoil in her refrigerator. Pushed far enough to stay put and plan a week's menu when she wanted to be out and about, she lost her temper and stormed out of the house. Within three months Bonnie confessed to Mrs. Pelham that Penny apparently did not want her help and gracefully bowed out. Penny had long since dropped out of night school. The attempt to transform her into a model middle-class woman thus came to a quiet and unofficial close.

In spite of the reported trouble in which the trust fund supporting Penny found itself, momentum toward selling the house gradually declined and Penny was left free to live as she pleased. Her case was eventually returned to Regional Center, at which time there was some suggestion of getting Penny into a sheltered workshop. But Penny was hardly aware of the services she might expect from her new counselor whom she had only seen once, and he, given a huge case load and myriad other responsibilities, was content to keep a very low profile. Penny continued to spend a great deal of time with her one female friend, Katy, an older woman (64), widowed with two children and three grandchildren, whom Mrs. Pelham described as being "like Penny but a little better". The two, who had met in the supermarket, wandered about town together to see their boyfriends, joined Katy's congregation for church picnics, ate out constantly, vacationed to San Diego occasionally, and, when they were sure her disapproving son would not stumble upon them, played with their dolls. Penny spent time alone as well, visiting her old pals at the bike shop, taking herself out for her birthday, or walking the neighborhood with her dog. Holidays, which in the past had been gala family affairs, were often lonely. The Davises refused to have her join them for holiday meals; either the Pelhams or neighbors would include her at the last moment on most occasions. But Penny continued to bask in the attention of men. While her accounts were sufficiently contradictory to reveal that some of the relationships in which she claimed to be involved contained elements of fantasy, she was clearly involved with a number of men, often more than one at the same time, though it was never clear which relationships were sexual and which platonic (as Penny declined to say and the eyes of Mrs. Pelham and other neighbors did not extend past the front door). In addition, Penny's list of acquaintances was endless — wherever she walked, she would meet someone she knew. But even in the face of this social activity, Penny left many — Mrs. Barnard, Mrs. Pelham, and her field researcher — suspecting that she was actually quite lonely.

For as long as Penny was able to maintain a relatively low profile, her relatives appeared to be content with the status quo. During the summer of 1978, however, Penny once again brought dramatic attention to herself: a man named Robert Prince, who had only recently taken up residence in Penny's home, died in her bed. While Penny was reluctant to reveal details of her relationship with this man, her friend Katy, who had heartily disapproved of him, was more than willing to comment. She had been with Penny the day she first encountered Prince outside of a department store. Penny had been attracted to his dog, and after making a big fuss over it, chatted about the kind of car Prince drove. When Penny expressed interest in seeing it, Prince offered to take Penny and Katy to a bar. Katy declined, unsettled by the man's scruffy appearance, but Penny accompanied him. A couple of days later, when Katy next chanced upon Penny, Prince had already moved all of his belongings into her house.

From her own house down the street, Mrs. Pelham observed the new man in Penny's life with disapproving eyes. He was another weird one, she felt, an ex-hippie to her eyes, with stringy dirty hair; moreover, he seemed dreadfully thin and pale, even sickly. She said and did nothing, however, watching silently as a truck pulled up to the house to cart away an old television and an antique desk which had belonged to Penny's father, hardly commenting when Penny explained that Prince's brakes needed some work and that she really didn't care about the items they had sold. When Penny later reported that Prince was experiencing severe stomach pains, Mrs. Pelham recommended the emergency room of a local hospital, though her suggestion wasn't followed. It became evident to Mrs. Pelham that Prince was in need of medical attention when he himself came over to her house to use her phone, and she took that occasion to advise him to see a doctor. She took no action, though, other than to inform the Davises of these events.

On July 10th, late in the afternoon, Penny ran over to a neighbor's house. Crying, she said that she thought Prince was dead. While the neighbor called the police, Mrs. Pelham entered the house to investigate and found Prince sprawled, spread-eagled, on the bed. He had violently hemorrhaged and there was blood all over the room. An investigator later revealed that Prince must have had cirrhosis of the liver. Judging by the state of the body, he had been spitting up black bile for a while and had probably died sometime during the preceding night, contradicting Penny's story that he had died while she was at the market. Prince, it seems, had told her he was going to die but warned her that he didn't want to go to the hospital or have anyone involved. "Just like an idiot", Penny later commented, "I didn't believe him. I should have."

Deciding once again that the house had to be sold and that Mrs. Pelham had been bearing a load that was not rightfully hers, the Davises bought a small trailer some 20 miles north of Penny's neighborhood into which they expected Penny to move by the beginning of August. Mrs. Pelham worried about Penny being isolated from people who would at least keep an eye on her. Laura, she indicated, expected that Penny's natural mother or grand-mother, both of whom lived near the trailer, would assume some responsi-bility for her. But these women, Mrs. Pelham knew, had neither the resources nor the desire to be involved with Penny. And Laura was equally reluctant to keep an eye on Penny; while she had assumed the role of trustee, she continually made it clear that was *not* a conservator. Mrs. Pelham, however, was tired of listening to the neighbors gossip about Penny parading nude around the house with the shades up or about the fact that the family plumber's son spent a half hour at the house when no plumbing problem had been reported. She was thus loathe to suggest that Penny remain in the neighborhood.

Seeking support for her plan to move Penny to a trailer, Laura contacted Penny's Regional Center counselor, about whom she had only recently learned — she had been under the impression that Penny's case had been closed for over a year. Dan, up to this point, had no knowledge of recent events in Penny's life. Laura explained that she and her parents had already taken Penny to see the trailer and reported her reaction as one of excitement and eagerness over the impending move. Penny had noted how nice it would be to move away from the nosey neighbors, Laura recounted, and had expressed no ambivalence over having to take her dog and cat to the pound. It was Laura's wish that Dan go to the house (to which he had never been, having met Penny only once before at breakfast) in order to see what had or hadn't been cleaned up, and that he take care of disposing the animals. He agreed to the first request but declined the second, in part because he suspected that regardless of what she had said, Penny would never willingly give up her animals. In spite of his suspicions, however, he made no plan to actually meet with Penny in order to ascertain her feelings on these major life changes. His feeling was that unless Penny called and directly asked for his assistance, there was no reason for him to get involved. If he happened upon Penny when he and the public health nurse made their visit — he planned on getting a key from Mrs. Pelham — he would talk to her then. But while he recognized that the relatives might be unfairly pressuring Penny into an unwanted move, he felt that advocacy on his part would be inappropriate unless requested by her. He had to assume that the family was concerned and acting in Penny's best interests, he said. If she missed her friends, animals, and neighborhood, that was simply something to which she would have to accustom herself.

Penny was, in fact, concerned over just these matters, though she wavered between wanting to remain where she was and wanting to acquiesce to her relatives' wishes. She confessed to the researcher that she was reluctant to live so far from the neighborhood and friends she knew so well, and was against the idea of taking her animals to the pound. She could understand the reasons for selling the house but questioned why the trailer could not be moved to a trailer park in the vicinity of her present home, preferably one that allowed pets. Nevertheless, she did recognize that her cousin Laura's attitude was unyielding. In the end, Penny felt it was futile to protest; she had no other choice but to resign herself to the idea of moving.

Concerned that to lift Penny out of the environment with which she was so familiar was both unfair and unnecessary, the researcher stepped out of her non-reactive role and arranged for a meeting between Penny and her counselor. By this time Dan had visited the house (though Penny, who *was* home at the time, had adamantly refused him and the public health nurse entry into the bedroom in which Prince had died). His conclusion, on the basis of what he had seen, was that Penny needed a more supervised living arrangement. But he remained reluctant about becoming involved and continued to put the onus on Penny. At breakfast, he reminded Penny that it was important that she tell him what she really wanted, and not what she felt other people wished. But he also told Penny that before he could act on her behalf, she had to call Laura and tell her personally that she neither wanted to give up the house nor move. "If she says, 'That's too bad, you're gonna do it anyway because we're gonna make you do it'", he continued, "then you can request me to help you. But I cannot call up Laura and say, 'No, you're not going to move Penny to this trailer'. You need to inform Laura first." Surprised by this statement, the researcher questioned whether Penny could stand up to Laura in that way. Dan offered that until she did so, his hands were tied. But, pointed out the researcher, before he had said that Penny had only to request his assistance. Now he was saying she had to confront Laura as well. Was that fair?

Penny's feelings on the move, meanwhile, were almost impossible to ascertain. As the tension rose between field researcher and counselor, she offered that perhaps it would be best for her to move, even if it did mean giving up her animals. Her natural grandmother (whom she had always claimed to detest) was out there, she pointed out, and she could always get other animals in the future. But later in the conversation she began to cry. She didn't want to call Laura but she didn't want to move. She wanted to stay where she was, with the friends, neighbors, and church that she knew. Still later, having calmed down, she returned to the idea of giving the move a try. "If I don't like it I can always move back. I just don't want to see my aunt and uncle [the Davises] anymore; that's why I was so upset. I just don't want them to come around anymore." Dan decided that unless Penny could tell him that she didn't want to move as adamantly as she had refused him entry into the room in which Prince had died, he would not contest the family's plans.

Because Laura was incapacitated by an injured knee, progress toward the move came to a temporary halt, giving Penny time to, as Mrs. Pelham put it, "go off again on another tangent". While at a picnic at the Veteran's Administration hospital with a new acquaintance, Joe, who was sour on her because she wouldn't "do it" with him, she met Eric Warner, a black Vietnam war veteran with a long history of psychiatric disturbance. Within days he moved all of his belongings into Penny's house and, according to Katy, began immediately taking charge of her allowance. Katy thought even less of Eric than she had of Prince — he was restless, nervous, on medication, sleepy-looking and clearly volatile; she feared what he might do were he to get angry. But Penny spoke fondly of him and began including him in her plans to move to the trailer.

In time, the move did occur. Shortly after Penny's birthday (which went unnoticed by all but a cousin at the bicycle shop), at the end of August, the Davises took sudden action. Burt Davis called Mrs. Pelham to inform her that Penny would be moved the following morning. Before then she was to both take her animals to the pound and pack a few things to temporarily hold her until they could decide what would fit in the 30 foot trailer. Penny said little when advised of this development but did comment when Mrs. Pelham indicated that Eric would not be permitted to join her, "He won't like that". Eric, in fact, stormed over to Mrs. Pelham's later in the day for a confrontation. Their two hour conversation, which later included Laura, extended over many topics. Most significantly, Eric cited Penny's reluctance to move, questioned their authority over her, and in a belligerent manner threatened them with lawyers; they, in turn, revealed that Penny was retarded, something which he had guessed but hadn't known for sure, and spoke frankly of her financial conditions in order to assure him that she would never have much. Informed of the upcoming move by the researcher, Dan chose not to be there the following morning, wanting to avoid a scene. He suggested that Penny, upon Laura's arrival, should tell her that she didn't want to move and then take the bus to his office — he would step in at that point. Penny did no such thing. She took her dog and cat to the pound, packed a few clothes, and, when Laura arrived to pick her up, closed the door of the house in which she had always lived.

Upon seeing Penny settled in the trailer and after making arrangements to send her weekly allowance, the Davises once again retired from the picture, leaving Eric free to join Penny. Since Eric had a car, living with him granted Penny a far greater degree of mobility, and she was thus able to return to her old haunts regularly, though always in his company. Eric's influence was not always a good one; their partnership held serious consequences for two of Penny's most secure and long-term relationships. Katy tired of the embarass-ing situations in which Eric placed her — borrowing money from the minister of her church and not repaying it, walking in and out during services, tripping the waitresses in the pancake restaurant, flashing a knife when the owner asked him to leave — and eventually chose to end their friendship. Mrs. Pelham also found Penny and Eric's visits disturbing. While she regretted letting Penny down, she eventually asked Laura to tell them that she no longer welcomed their company.

January 1979 found Penny contemplating a new change — a move with Eric to New York, where his family lived. Totally committed to the idea,

Penny became furious if Eric or anyone else tried to suggest that January was perhaps not the most propitious time of year for a cross-country trek. Pushed to explain why it was so important for her to get away, Penny finally revealed that that year's Christmas had irrevocably confirmed for her the extent to which her family had rejected her. With the exception of Mrs. Pelham, who had sent her two dollars, and her cousin from the bicycle shop, she had been remembered by no one. A long roster of relatives, from the Davises to another aunt and uncle in the vicinity who had shunned her for years to her natural mother and grandmother who only barely acknowledged her when she would pass them on the street, were earmarked as individuals with no regard for her feelings whatsoever. She wanted nothing more to do with any of them, and moving three thousand miles away was an effective means toward that end. Inured to Penny's life style by this time and relieved by the thought of her absence, Laura gave Penny her blessing and, more importantly, money for the trip, arranging for Penny to receive an allowance regularly once she became settled in New York. The trailer was sold and Penny left the West coast.

Penny was not received in New York with completely open arms. Eric's mother was quick to realize that Penny was handicapped and offered, during a phone conversation, that Eric did not need another liability at this point in his life — if he had to be hospitalized, she wondered, who would look after Penny. Later conversations revealed her continuing concern. She reiterated her feeling that Eric should not have brought Penny to New York and her frustration over Penny's refusal to take proper care of herself. Eric too was not without second thoughts. Penny, he felt, held him back from going out alone, cussing him and his friends if they attempted to leave their basement apartment without her. Moreover, he didn't feel comfortable leaving her alone as she had already become too friendly with the men in the neighborhood. Confessing that he was "a little disgusted with Penny", he indicated that he was contemplating sending her back to Los Angeles. If Penny was aware of the qualms of her man and her "in-laws", she gave no indication of it. She loved New York, she claimed, and was already getting to know the neighborhood and its inhabitants.

Different reports filtered in from the East coast during the next few months: Eric was in jail briefly on a drug-related charge; Penny was getting along well with all of Eric's family except one sister; Eric was enrolled in a small, private music school; Penny and Eric had to move because of an argument between Eric and the landlord; Eric had left school and was considering a job driving a cab. Amidst all of the ups and downs, however, Eric continued to return to the possibility of sending Penny back home. He spent much, even most, of his time with Penny, he said, which thrilled her but bored him. "I look at what I could have done and see what I got", he said in the beginning of May, a sentiment which did not bode well for the future.

On May 14, Eric put Penny on a plane for Los Angeles with enough money for food and lodging for a couple of days. Calling the researcher so that someone would know she was arriving, he explained that he had reached the end of his patience with Penny and had decided that she was "more or less a liability". Mrs. Warner, adding her opinion, complained that Penny was dirty, refused to take care of herself or her house, and was uninterested in changing. Moreover, she was a liar and a trouble maker. "We all tried to accept her", she concluded, "but she's man hungry. We cautioned her not to make trouble but trouble seems to be her middle name." Eric felt sorry that he and Penny had not been able to make a go of it but offered, in a very telling statement, "She can find somebody else . . . to give her money to. It just didn't work out."

Laura gave a brief, wry laugh when contacted by the field researcher with the news of Penny's impending arrival and said that she had been expecting this. She confirmed, however, that the trailer and house had both been sold and resolved that the family would neither meet Penny's plane nor welcome her into their own homes. She agreed to call the Regional Center at the suggestion of the field researcher but only after reminding her in an utterly frank tone that "my responsibility is with the money. No one is legally responsible for Penny's life."

Dan's reaction to Laura's call was by this time predictable — there was nothing he could do until Penny called him and made a direct request for services. He reassured Laura (who needed little reassurance) that Penny was resourceful and knew the bus system well. There was no doubt in his mind that she would take care of herself. To the field researcher he reiterated that Penny was not helpless, and that finding an apartment or other lodging was not a service which Regional Center provided. He suggested that if the field researcher heard from Penny, she should recommend that she get in touch with him. Finally, he confessed that had he known that Penny had moved to New York, he would have closed her case.

Penny did call the researcher the following day and revealed that she had indeed been resourceful. She had spent the preceding evening in a motel with "this other dude" whom she had met on the bus from the airport. She had stopped by the bicycle shop to get some money from her cousin there but needed to find a more permanent place to stay. Breaking into tears, she sobbed that she still loved Eric but now found herself in love with this guy Pete (whose last name she couldn't remember). He wanted her to go to Mexico with him and while the idea was enticing, she was bothered both by a lingering feeling of loyalty to Eric and a fear of drinking the Mexican water. Moreover, Pete was on drugs, though she was sure she could quickly cure him of that. Money, for the moment, was not a problem; Penny reassured her that she had "two tens, two twenties, and some ones".

For two months, Penny lived in a series of motels, staying at each for a couple of weeks until the manager requested that she leave, either because they had supposedly promised the room or because she had become too familiar with the other guests. Her cousin at the bicycle shop, and then Dan, assumed responsibility for doling out money to her, though as per Laura's new policy, Penny was now free to ask for and spend as much as she pleased. (Dan suspected that the family was anxious to see the trust fund totally depleted so that they could be completely free from any responsibility for Penny.) Eventually Dan, having exhausted his list of potential semi-independent residential facilities and tired of his futile attempts to have Penny turn in receipts for all of her expenditures, convinced Laura to pay for an occupational therapist to locate an apartment for Penny.

By the end of August, Karen, a former special education teacher hired by Dan, had found Penny a small one bedroom apartment in a low income area a few miles from her old neighborhood. Dan prevailed upon Laura to place Penny on an allowance again and together they decided she would receive $30 on Mondays and $45 on Fridays for food and entertainment; Laura took care of paying the rent and utilities. Meanwhile, Karen convinced Laura that Penny would profit by having someone see her on a regular basis and act as a trouble shooter. Laura agreed, and Karen began seeing Penny about every five days, sometimes just to go out to lunch and chat, other times to take care of such practical matters as buying clothes, obtaining medical care, getting haircuts, shopping for household items. Karen did try to influence Penny's choice of men for a time, fearing for her safety. Penny's response was to refuse to see her for several months. Karen thus learned not to impose her values on Penny's life-style, and as a result, the two of them got along tolerably well.

Penny ostensibly found it easy to adapt to her new living environment, as different and full of trials as it was. Her apartment was located in a predominantly commercial area of town on a street lined with ethnic fast food places and populated largely by black, hispanic, and oriental individuals. The neighborhood contained more than its fair share of drug addicts and alcoholics and violence was a common occurrence. Penny's initiation into this violence took place almost immediately. On her first weekend in her new home she invited two strangers into her apartment. They, in turn, invited five of their friends, and left only after getting Penny drowsy with beer, molesting her, and lifting her wallet and bus pass. Later in the year, a man who had previously lived with her for a brief period of time kicked in her door, leaving a large crack down the middle. Still later, a brick was thrown through her window, nearly striking a couple seated on the couch — Penny's current *beau* and his friend took after the perpetrators with a knife. Penny confessed that the police and fire departments were regular visitors to her apartment.

During this time, Penny was not without her boyfriends. In addition to those mentioned above, Jackson, a bus driver she had known in the past, reappeared with promises to take her to Arkansas; Paul charmed her with plans of marriage and a trip out of town; a drug addict from across the way would occasionally ask for and receive permission to spend the night. At the same time, Penny busied herself with the affairs of all her neighbors, continually visited her favorite hang-outs (often running into Katy, who continued to studiously ignore her), sporadically dropped in on Mrs. Pelham (who was less firm in her resolve than Katy), and blithely allowed life to carry her along in her characteristically unconcerned fashion.

September, 1980, found Penny contemplating life's bitter and sweet sides. She had found herself a new man several weeks before, a black construction worker, aged 48, by the name of J. J. While they were not yet married, a date had been set, and Penny, in anticipation of the event, already referred to him as her husband, his grown children as her children, his friends as her friends. She was terribly preoccupied with plans for the wedding and a honeymoon trip to Oklahoma with a band to which J. J. belonged. She paid far less attention to the fact that the door to her apartment had been completely shattered by a previous acquaintance who had been looking for money. Likewise it was of secondary importance to her that she had received an eviction notice, the result (according to Karen) of both the constant arguments in which she engaged with neighbors and the steady stream of men who had passed through her apartment. Despite the fact that the eviction date was rapidly approaching, Penny was only desultorily searching for alternative living arrangements. Laura, she knew, was aware of the eviction because the manager had returned the second rent check. Penny thus assumed that she, or Karen, or someone, would find her a place to live when the time came for her to leave.

Penny was ultimately, but not immediately, correct in her assumption. The day J. J. and Penny had to leave her apartment arrived before a place had been found — even before anyone had begun to search. Left without a place, they camped out on the floor of an abandoned warehouse which J. J. had known about until Laura provided money for a motel a week later. Karen was recruited to apartment hunt again and was finally successful in the beginning of November. Penny and J. J. took up residence in a small, furnished apartment in a low income but far more respectable neighborhood.

While plans to marry never came to fruition, J. J. and Penny did remain together for some time. J. J. was often affectionate and did keep Penny well fed. But he was a man who could get nasty when he drank and who would occasionally hit her. Moreover, he retained the right to come and go as he pleased, leaving Penny wondering where he was as many times as informing her of his whereabouts and time of return. He faithfully accompanied her on Fridays to pick up her check from Dan — Penny was by this point receiving $85 once a week — but would invariably take off for the weekend with a good deal of the money, explaining that the band had a gig and that no "wives" were invited. And while he insisted on the freedom to do so, he became enraged if he returned home from a weekend party unannounced and didn't find Penny at home, accusing her of seeing other men.

Penny was not without company when J. J. was out entertaining himself

Ted has grown more preoccupied with the prospect of locating a girl whose name he does not recall. What he does remember is that "when I was in school (post-hospitalization), she keeps looking at me all the time".

Whenever I picked my eyes up she was lookin'. We would all the time get together. Walk around, go to the show together, go out uh, then we go places; I just, uh anything to kill time.

But taken out of the Burbank Schools to work in 1944, Ted lost track of her. With similar misfortune, Ted notes the disappearance of an extraordinarily beautiful woman who, according to fellow employees of a bar in the early 1960s, dropped by to see Ted, waited for him, and then left forever before he could return from an errand. Josephine also remains elusive, a woman with whom Ted briefly cohabited but from whom he only felt hints of her feeling toward him. "She wouldn't go out and tell you or nothin'. We was necking several times. Didn't both me anyway." Ted's transience has probably determined much of his isolation from these figures. "You lose things, like address books. I had lots of good numbers, but I lost 'em all."

Casual acquaintances fill much of Ted's social time, relationships in which Ted seems to maintain joking contact but makes little additional commitment. In fact, the commitment is usually directed toward Ted from these others. Tim, for example, used to be a regular companion on trips on Tijuana where they would sleep on the bar benches of a bar owning friend of Tim's. The proprietor's death precipitated less cordial reception for the weekends, so Tim now reminds Ted of the good times that even in memory keep their relationship strong. Tim now urges Ted to apply for subsidized housing and become a neighbor; there's a loneliness about Tim's fond attentions which speaks of how much he would like that to happen. Lyle, who lives upstairs in Ted's hotel, has made a number of public and private overtures for Ted's sexual attentions, open as he is to such occasional sexual play, Ted openly acts his "girl-boy" routine and dismisses Lyle's pressure with public descriptions of Lyle as his "Oo-oo mother, my roto-rooter!" Grant nervously solicits Ted in his room to find a whore who will fulfill Grant's sexual needs for free. Ted is disparaging in his advice: "What's the use of taking them out if you can't afford to take a girl out to a good steak dinner?"

Two strong relationships he maintains are characterized by Ted in terms of the dependency needs of the women involved. These relationships are not extensions of the boldly spirited, and public, whimsy which Ted daily casts in the direction of Gordon's Restaurant waitresses. The latter suffer his grasps and mischievous howls as if they've figured out that this is the guy who years before, as a member of a friendship club set up for former mental hospital residents living in the city, scrupulously avoided any serious competition for desirable females.

Tim counsels Ted to terminate his friendship with Judy, a former burlesque dancer whose naked torso drapes suggestively across a post card wedged along the edge of Ted's bureau mirror. Ted bemoans his presumed manage the job's demands. But near the park, where daily life can be very routine, there is still the unpredictable occasional situation which stimulates Ted's good sense for deft evasion. Ted accepts as pivotal to his life the savvy in knowing how and when to back off. In the country, he's not so sure that ranch living would not be, in its routine isolation, unbearably predictable. As Ted pointedly puts it, "What are you going to do, screw the horses?"

FRIENDSHIP AND THE BENEFACTOR ROLE

One of Ted's great disappointments of late has been the police surveillance, and therefore *de facto* curfews, which have dispersed flourishing friendships among transients and loiterers in the park. Under such pressure, many of Ted's friends have filtered away from the area, and Ted finds himself enjoying trips to the park less and less. Increasingly, despite his frequent urban odysseys, Ted notes that "what few friends I got are from the hospital", those whom he either knew there as a teen-ager or has come to know as former patients of the institution.

Aw, some people I do know from the hospital, yea. I go in, tell the (clerk); I know him. Then he goes and does what he wants. You know, then I just go back in the laundimat (*sic*) and see what I have to do there.

Such meetings of former patients are usually serendipitous however, and are flavored by the shared recognition that a mutual incarceration will likely foster a continual passing in and out of each other's lives. Friendships with staff at the Department of Mental Hygiene (now the Department of Mental Health), upon which Ted had grown dependent from 1944 to 1957, were summarily concluded at official discharge from hospital roles. Since that time, Ted has "been afraid to go down there ever since I been released".

They just laughed at me. I told some of the social workers; shit, they just laughed at me. "Get the hell out of the goddamn place." I go to the office and they just laugh at me and they just close the door in my face and I walk out.

One of these staff members did however prove integral to facilitating Ted's acceptance for State disability benefits in the early seventies; a fondness she felt for Ted remained from a relationship long before officially severed. Nevertheless, for Ted, the friendships of those years deteriorated at an unreasonable rate and he has never fully reconciled himself to that shift.

For the present, Ted occupies himself with dreams of relationships that might have been, or could still be, with lost female friends; he engages in an array of relationships with males who cluster around the restaurant or are co-residents of the hotel, and he devotes considerable energy to long-term relations with women for whom he envisions himself as a sustaining bene-factor.

Penny's chosen life-style assaulted their values, combined with their natural reluctance to assume complete responsibility for Penny, made them less than satisfactory replacements. Within a short time, all but Mrs. Pelham withdrew from any contact with Penny whatsoever and even Mrs. Pelham, burdened as she was with her own problems, tended to observe, rather than participate in Penny's life. The Davises somewhat unwillingly met their commitment to administer the trust fund but it was only because of this responsibility that they remained even indirectly bound to Penny. They made it quite clear that they would not involve themselves directly with her regardless of the circumstances — they were responsible for the money, as Laura said, and not for her life. All social amenities eventually disappeared, and the relationship settled into a contractual one only: they would see that Penny's most basic needs of food, clothing, and shelter were provided for but their responsibility ended there. This is not to say they exerted no influence on Penny's life. Indeed, at those times when their *laissez faire* policy lapsed, their decisions stood as testaments to the power they held to radically alter her existence as they saw fit.

In addition to Penny's relatives, members of the service delivery system walked in and out of Penny's life subsequent to her father's death, playing different roles at different times. Eloise Barnard and Bonnie were eager to play a crucial role in Penny's life. Unfortunately, the role they chose for themselves was not one which Penny was willing to accept. Rather than live her life as a pristine middle-class matron, she opted to alienate them. In fact, she was fully aware of all they wanted to teach her — how to cook, how to clean, how to groom herself, how to shop — but she preferred to do otherwise. No affective ties bound Mrs. Barnard or Bonnie to Penny. Thus, when she made it clear she would not play the game according to their rules, they felt free to withdraw from her life.

Dan was far less eager to play a central role; if anything, he constantly dodged available opportunities to intervene and advocate on Penny's behalf, maintaining that steps which other Regional Center counselors had readily taken in similar situations were not part of his job. While he was more realistic than his predecessors in not trying to impose his values on Penny, his motivation for doing so seemed to relate more to a desire to avoid involvement than a careful consideration of the issues. In the end, the service delivery system failed to produce the kind of individual who might have had some impact: an individual who knew Penny well, who was sensitive to her idiosyncracies (i.e. who realized that the fact that she was able to refuse Dan entry into her bedroom did not mean she could as readily confront Laura with her desire not to move), who respected her chosen life-style, and who with her best interests at heart could act on Penny's behalf.

While not actually part of the delivery system, Karen has most closely approximated this role — she has been someone who could, as she says, "trouble shoot", making sure that Penny's medical needs have been met, providing a resource to which Penny could turn in an emergency, and lending Penny advice when she has sought it. The fact remains, however, that Karen has played this role because she has been paid by the trust and not because of more durable feelings of loyalty to Penny, much in the same way that field researchers have been involved with Penny because it is part of their jobs. Should circumstances change in Karen's life or should the trust show signs of insolvency, her involvement would abruptly end.[3]

Penny's current support system, then, does contain a stable core of individuals who have consistently met her basic financial needs (the Davises and her cousin at the bicycle shop) and other practical needs (Karen). These individuals, however, do not accept responsibility for satisfying Penny's more affective needs for love, companionship, and day-to-day emotional as well as utilitarian support. For this, Penny looks to the friends, acquaintances, and lovers she so relentlessly pursues and who so quickly pass through her life. But her friends and acquaintances (the latter far outnumbering the former) are tied to her by only the loosest of bonds, and while she can rely on them for conversation, bus fare, or even small favors, they do not in any sense constitute a group upon which she can securely depend over time. Her lovers are only slightly more reliable — while the prospects of Penny's apartment and allowance, as well as her warmth and compliance, attract them readily enough, they do tend to be drifters, do tire of her, and do move on. Thus the segment of Penny's support system from which she seeks the satisfaction of her social and emotional needs consists of unstable, shifting, impermanent and largely superficial relationships. Her emotional support largely lies in the hands of relative strangers and others who are in no substantial way committed to her. Such support, superficial as it is, can easily be left behind and readily replaced elsewhere. As a result, Penny's life is constantly in flux, as shifting and unstable as the relationships within it. It is perhaps in the poverty of the dependable emotional support available to her that the consequences of her father's death are most readily apparent.

As tempting as it is to view Penny as an unfortunate victim leading an unenviable existence, to do so would not be faithful to Penny's own perception of her current life, as far as that perception can be determined. A life dictated by the rules and conventions so highly touted by her relatives, Eloise Barnard, and Bonnie might have been more safe and stable but it was not the life of her choosing. Penny's boundless curiosity about other people, her need to get out, mingle with them, and even bring them into her home and bed was far more important to her. Moreover, Penny has given no indication that she views her life with the alarm which these and other middle-class, settled, security-conscious minds do. Many would point to her relationships with her lovers as being shamefully exploitative, for instance. Were she to give it any thought, she would undoubtedly reject the idea, and in fact her relationships may be less parasitic than they appear. Penny does end up turning over a good deal of money to her man, does endure a double standard, and does occasionally suffer physical abuse. She receives in exchange, however, the company and care of a mate, even if temporarily, as well as the emotional security that comes from being able to proclaim that she is one half of a couple.

But the point is that Penny does not really give any thought to the issue of whether her lovers are taking advantage of her. And while others living Penny's life might be devastated by the threat of personal danger which she often faces, the dearth of real emotional support available to her, her tenuous financial security, the lack of guarantees which life holds for her, and her basic powerlessness, Penny unquestioningly lives each day as it comes, thinking little of the past and even less of the future. Blissfully non-introspective, she buries or sanitizes tragedies and threatening situations, ignores the slights of those who choose not to tolerate her overtures, rolls with life's punches and simply carries on. This is not to say that she has no feelings. On more than one occasion she has referred to her confusion over her family's rejection of her and her wish that it could be otherwise. It is to say that her practice of not defining certain situations as being upsetting or threatening, her vague acceptance of everything that happens, her willingness to be carried along by life's current, together function as a highly effective coping mechanism which serves to ameliorate the damaging consequences her flimsy emotional support system might hold for someone more sensitive, more future-oriented, more prone to worrying. Her thick skin, unshakeable faith in other people, lack of self-consciousness, and generally unreflective attitude toward life allow her to pass through tumultuous events and day-to-day stresses seemingly unaffected.

In a word, Penny is a survivor. She has weathered the death of her parents and the radical changes which eventually followed, the rejection of her relatives, a gruesome experience with a dying boyfriend, a series of affairs, one of which took her as far as New York, the violence of neighborhoods quite unlike those in which she was raised, and passage through untold numbers of transient relationships. Further, she gives every indication that she will continue to adjust to whatever circumstances in which she finds herself. Her future is virtually impossible to predict. Penny will travel which ever way the wind blows her, especially if the trust fund expires. But she *will* survive, resourcefully finding someone to look after and care for her, and then someone else, and then someone else. As time goes by, her life will undoubtedly resemble less and less the one she lived as a child and young adult. But Penny, it seems, will cope with whatever comes, without measuring it against what she has had or will have, tacitly accepting her life as it is.

CONCLUSION

What, then, can Penny's life history tell us about social support and support systems? Above all else, Penny's experiences call attention to the fact that support systems are dynamic entities which constantly change over both long and short periods of time. A diachronic and processual framework is thus a necessary complement to current synchronic approaches. While important in their own right, synchronic studies cannot incorporate the ever-shifting nature of support systems, and the way they affect and are affected by unfolding life circumstances. Yet the very flux which static approaches tend to obscure holds the promise of contributing vastly to our understanding of the relationship between social support and individual adaptation. For it is in examining change and observing how changes in support systems affect the quality of life and well-being of individuals that the impact of social support on individual adaptation can be most blatantly revealed. Adaptation, it must be remembered, is by definition a process involving continual alteration and adjustment over time. It would thus seem to make sense to embrace the flux which is such an enduring characteristic of support systems and to discover what that flux can tell us, rather than restricting ourselves to approaches which barely acknowledge its existence.

If there is a second lesson to be learned from Penny's experiences, it is that the impact of social support on an individual's adaptation cannot be completely understood if social support is viewed exclusively as a phenomenon which exists external to the individual. While one can isolate the constituent elements of an individual's support system, measure it in some way and manipulate it as a variable, to do so and to feel that its full impact on an individual has been approximated is to impute a passivity and a *tabula rasa* quality to people which simply does not exist. In reality, the impact of available social support is to a large degree dependent on how it is individually and subjectively mediated. In order to fully understand the impact which an individual's support system has on his or her general adaptation and well-being, we must attend to the meaning it holds for that individual — to the very subjective way in which that individual perceives it. Similarly, we must know how that individual defines her needs, what it takes for her to feel that they are satisfied, and how she defines the situations in which she finds herself. A support system, in other words, must be viewed not only as a social reality but as a psychological reality as well, especially if one's purpose is to delineate the way in which support ameliorates the consequences of stress and contributes to well-being.

All of this is to say that the actual process by which people derive support from the social world in which they live is an extraordinarily complex one. Methods which freeze support systems in time and which represent them solely through the use of predetermined, quantifiable variables can only tell us so much. Alternative approaches — ones which attend to the changing behavior and circumstances of people in context and over time, and which focus on the meaning which people lend to and extract from the world in which they live — will go a long way toward enriching our appreciation of issues related to social support and individual adaptation.

ACKNOWLEDGEMENT

The preparation of this paper was made possible by the Mental Retardation Research Center, University of California at Los Angeles (USPHS Grant HD-04612-05), the Community Context of Normalization Study (NICHD Grant HD-09474-02), and by the Community Adaptation of Mildly Retarded Persons Study (USPHS 5 PO1 HD11944). I gratefully acknowledge the research assistance of Marsha Bollinger, Lorel Cornman, and Linda Hubbard.

NOTES

1. When Bob Davis died, his brother, in order to prove Penny's eligibility for Social Security benefits, had taken her to a psychiatrist who had recommended that he contact the Kennedy Regional Center for the Developmentally Disabled. (Surviving children of adult age cannot receive benefits from their parents unless it is shown that they are disabled dependents.) Penny had thus been a client of the Regional Center for almost a year, though in that time she had received no direct services and had not been seen by a counselor subsequent to intake.
2. It was at this point that a field researcher first began visiting Penny.
3. The trust, it should be pointed out, stands as one constant in Penny's life since her father's death that should not be ignored in any consideration of Penny's support system. Because of what her father bequeathed her, and because of the manner in which her relatives have arranged her affairs, Penny's rent and utilities are automatically paid and she is guaranteed, at least for now, $85 per week. Moreover, money from the trust pays for Karen's services, Penny's medical care, her clothing, etc. Should the trust run out of money, Penny would not be destitute — she would still have her Social Security Survivor benefits and would be eligible for both Supplemental Security Income (SSI) and Medi-Cal. She would receive these sums only once a month, however, and would be personally responsible for both paying her bills and budgeting her money (as her relatives would undoubtedly withdraw completely in such an event). As it is, Penny is chronically broke three days after she has received her check. Her prospects for having to manage her money on a monthly basis would not appear to be good.

REFERENCES

Basham, R.
    1978 *Urban anthropology.* Palo Alto, CA: Mayfield Publishing Co.
Cassel, J.
    1974 An epidemiological perspective of psychosocial factors in disease etiology. *American Journal of Public Health, 64*: 1040—1043.
Cassel, J.
    1975 Social science in epidemiology: Psychosocial processes and "stress" theoretical formulation. *In* E. L. Struening and M. Guttentag (eds.), *Handbook of evaluation research* (Vol. 1). Beverly Hills: Sage Publications.
Clark, M.
    1970 *Health in the Mexican-American culture.* Berkeley: University of California Press.
Cobb, S.
    1976 Social support as a moderator of life stress. *Psychosomatic Medicine, 38*: 300—314.
Cohen, C. I. and Sokolovsky, J.
    1978 Schizophrenia and social networks: Ex-patients in the inner city. *Schizophrenia Bulletin, 4*: 546—560.

Crapanzano, V.
    1973 *The Hamadsha. A study of Moroccan ethnopsychiatry.* Berkeley: University of
          California Press.
Dean, A. and Lin, N.
    1977 Stress-buffering role of social support: Problems and prospects for systematic
          investigation. *Journal of Nervous and Mental Disease, 165*: 403—417.
Finlayson, A.
    1976 Social networks as coping resources. *Social Science and Medicine, 10*: 97—103.
Fox, J. R.
    1964 Witchraft and clanship in Cochiti therapy. *In* Ari Kiev (ed.), *Magic, faith, and
          healing.* New York: The Free Press.
Freed, S. A. and Freed, R. S.
    1964 Spirit possession as illness in a north Indian village. *Ethnology, 3*: 152—171.
Froland, C., Brodsky, G., Olson, M. and Stewart, L.
    1979 Social support and social adjustment: Implications for mental health professionals.
          Community Mental Health Journal, 15: 82—93.
Garrison, V.
    1978 Support systems of schizophrenic and non-schizophrenic Puerto Rican migrant
          women in New York City. *Schizophrenia Bulletin, 4*: 561—596.
Gelein, J. L.
    1980 The aged American female: Relationships between social support and health.
          Journal of Gerontological Nursing, 6: 69—73.
Gore, S.
    1978 The effect of social support in moderating the health consequences of unemploy-
          ment. *Journal of Health and Social Behavior, 19*: 157—165.
Gulick, J.
    1974 Urban anthropology. *In* J. Honigmann (ed.), *The handbook of social and cultural
          anthropology.* Chicago: Rand McNally.
Hammer, M., Makiesky-Barrow, S. and Gutwirth, L.
    1978 Social networks and schizophrenia. *Schizophrenia Bulletin, 4*: 522—545.
Henderson, S.
    1977 Do support systems prevent psychiatric disorders? *Medical Journal of Australia, 1*:
          622—664.
Kaplan, R. H., Cassel, J. C. and Gore, S.
    1977 Social support and health. *Medical Care, 15*: 471—482, supp.
Kennedy, J. G.
    1967 Nubian Zar ceremonies as psychotherapy. *Human Organization, 26*: 185—194.
Koegel, P.
    1982 Rethinking support systems: A qualitative investigation into the nature of social
          support. Unpublished doctoral dissertation.
Langness, L. L.
    1965 *The life history in anthropological science.* New York: Holt, Rinehart and Winston.
Langness, L. L. and Frank, G.
    1981 *Lives: An anthropological approach to biography.* Novato, CA: Chandler and Sharp.
Lewis, I. M.
    1966 Spirit possession and deprivation cults. *Man, 1*: 307—329.
Lin, N., Ensel, W. M., Simeone, R. S. and Kuo, W.
    1973 Social support, stressful life events, and illness: A model and an empirical test.
          Journal of Health and Social Behavior, 20: 108—119.
Lopata, H. Z.
    1975 Support systems of elderly urbanites: Chicago of the 1970s. *The Gerontologist,
          15*(1): 35—41.

Lowenthal, H. F. and Haven, C.
 1968 Interaction and adaptation: Intimacy as a critical variable. *American Sociological Review, 33*: 20—30.
Nuckolls, K., Cassel, J. and Kaplan B.
 1972 Psychosocial assets, life crisis, and the prognosis of pregnancy. *American Journal of Epidemiology, 95*: 431—441.
Pattison, E. M., DeFrancisco, D., Wood, P., Frazier, H. and Crowder, J.
 1975 A psychosocial kinship model for family therapy. *American Journal of Psychiatry, 132*(12): 1246—1251.
Pilisuk, M. and Froland, C.
 1978 Kinship, social networks, social support and health. *Social Science and Medicine, 12B*: 273—280.
Snyder, P. Z.
 1976 Neighborhood gatekeepers in the process of urban adaptation: Cross-ethnic commonalities. *Urban Anthropology, 5*(1): 35—52.
Turner, V.
 1964 An Ndembu doctor in practice. *In* Ari Kiev (ed.), *Magic, faith, and healing*. New York: The Free Press.
Walker, K. M., MacBride, A. and Vachon, M. L. A.
 1977 Social support networks and the crisis of bereavement. *Social Science and Medicine, 11*: 35—41.
Wan, T. H.
 1982 *Stressful life events, social support networks, and gerontological health*. Lexington, MA: Lexington Books.
Winefield, H. R.
 1979 Social support and the social environment of depressed and normal women. *Australian and New Zealand Journal of Psychiatry, 13*: 335—339.

ROBERT D. WHITTEMORE

THEODORE V. BARRETT:
AN ACCOUNT OF ADAPTIVE COMPETENCE

INTRODUCTION

His weary head reclined so as to ease the cigar's smoke about the room, Theodore Barrett piles ashes in a saucer brimming with gray flakes. On two holiday visits this year, when he will exchange his single-occupancy hotel room for familial companionship in his sister's home in Anaheim, Ted will take along a sack of these ashes. They are good for her roses; nor will he forget the coins, sorted and rolled to fill a bulging pocket, which her children gratefully accept from their "Uncle Teddy".

He won't be long away from the Los Angeles street grid, the deteriorating park area enclave in which he is a longstanding resident. In the latter portion of his fifty years, he finds his ease in this extraordinary urban landscape. His personal map of it is marked with the street coordinates of liquor stores and laundromats which have afforded him occasional employment, the hang-outs of pick-pockets, "queens", and those practicing the anomalous lives of urban confusion, and where inner-city wanderers group together in empty lots, on brownstone entrances, around sidewalk vendors. His sagging mattress in the middle of it all is his retreat, surrounded by his chamber's surfeit of found and donated objects. Here, with dwindling cigars, ashes flaking onto his expansive belly, he thinks about the world outside his room and door.

Ted has never believed that talking to oneself was a problem. For him it is just a part of thinking. The danger sign, he feels, is when the walls start "answering". But they never have for Ted. He watches out for that. Out loud, he reflects on Gordon's Restaurant[1] and its short order cook and the whiz-kid who washes dishes instead of going to college, the open-air Public Market downtown and its once foot-long hot dogs, the social security system and a price of living increase, or a miserable heat wave and the inadequacies of a small electric fan. His present life and his past history are wrapped up in these visions. These are not senescent reminiscences cast back over a wide arc of life. They are repeated conjurings for himself, and for me, and in their telling they incorporate an array of happenings, shared experiences, and personal passages which explain, and daily help him effect, his continuing life's management.

The life account which Ted chooses to present is the one he carries with him from day to day, privately or publicly declaring aspects of it for a variety of reasons, casting them up against the vagaries of his present circumstances. For despite past familial estrangement, a severe accident at the age of five years, institutionalization, prolonged hospital parole, and

155

L. L. Langness and H. G. Levine (eds.), Culture and Retardation, 155—189.
© 1986 *by D. Reidel Publishing Company.*

life-long inability to maintain lasting employment, Theodore V. Barrett, like Penny in the previous account (Koegel, this volume), is a survivor.

As he continues to approach life with his share of critical incidents, those which he continues to present may indeed correspond to those available in official records, recollections of his siblings, and views of his street-life friends. From such sources, Ted Barrett's life account resembles that of other individuals presumed "retarded" at an early age: socio-economic hardship in the family, instability of parental relations, familial transience, personal early isolation from the family unit, devastating contact with the social service delivery system, and ultimately a resigned helplessness to the consequences of that past and the designs of service personnel motivated by that documented personal history.

However, Ted's own recollection of much of what is in this record is usually foggy. To honor the overlap as well as the discrepancy between documented history and Ted's self-presentation is one task of this discussion. To make available Ted's past, even as he allows it to emerge spontaneously in his daily life course, is another.

"STUFF I LIKE TO WATCH"

As part of an effort to have Ted expound upon his daily life, a previous researcher[2] procured a super-eight camera and film for him. After we viewed for the first time what Ted broadly described as "stuff I like to watch", I asked him if someone could learn something about Ted Barrett's life from the movie.

I guess they would, what I do. I shoot of what I shoot of. I like to shoot, what I like to do. Well, maybe, maybe everybody doesn't like what, don't like to, do like I do: go here or go there. I do about what everybody else does, just go where you want to go. So I just, shoot and go; or go down to the park and talk to my friends, or I see my friends, we're talking, shooting the bull, or I go downtown and you walk around, or go home and listen to the music. I watch T.V. or go to my brother's house and see him.

With surprising lack of reactivity to his task, thinking of the sweep of his camera as but an extension of his usual perambulations, he makes an apologia to those who might not see things quite as he does. But, he makes it clear, this is a personal presentation of his world as he would see it, "do" in it, and join in the stream of individuals who are part of it.

Viewing his efforts, Ted heavily criticized his own technical proficiency. He devotes several long segments of film to the late-night filming of an *FBI Story* episode, on location, on a downtown street. The running and re-running of a vintage FBI-versus-gangster auto chase rivets Ted's lens, but he was vexed that his version had not mirrored televised cinematographic technique. Ted finds no aesthetic appeal in unfocused headlights passing toward, and sweeping under, his lens as he stands above the Harbor

Freeway. He complains that he has not caught the scene as it really is. He does not measure up to his expectations of what he was sure he could catch. At a later date, when I remarked on what I sincerely took to be some remarkable film shooting, Ted grew more irritated than I have ever witnessed him to be. He could only interpret my praise as aimed to barb his self-perceived incompetence.

By his standards, other shots, or "old-time" cars and trains at an amusement park and a steady and deliberate scan of the oldest street in Los Angeles, are worthy. Ted and I have walked Los Angeles streets, guided by history's changes which he points out: the site of a funicula which, for ten cents, transported him on countless occasions to the top of Bunker Hill before Government Center urban renewal scheduled its razing; the old theatres whose signs' rust and deterioration he bemoans as the years of their shining brilliance fade in the city's memory. These are highly personal symbols of the past. Whether scanning Elliott Ness's Hollywood car chase, or an invisible funicula, or the once bright lights of downtown, Ted attempts to retrieve the context for his own past history.

Indeed, observing what has changed, "what's different" as he puts it, is often his motivation for exploring the city; he spots with little apparent effort the variability in a very confusing landscape. In the park, which is the hub of the urban neighborhood of which he is a member, his film emphasizes the bizarre. From the park's summer stage, Ted finds disorienting the motivation of a Sunday preacher's oration or the musical prowess of a playing trombonist simultaneously bowing a violin with his trombone slide. But such things are documented by the film; these regular park performers' idiosyncrasies warrant their inclusion in the park scene. He comments on the aesthetics of numerous things: the mock combat from a Shakespeare-in-the-Park production, the camera's pursuit of the skyscraping thrust of City Hall and its horizontal aerial walkway, the miniature marvels of Knott's Berry Farm dioramas, and a glass menagerie window display. Just as his keen eye sees the details, so his camera dwells on them.

Ted takes us to settings which fill his routine: the restaurant in which he eats, the liquor store in which he once worked and then quit because of the miserable pay. In the store, though he was on his last roll of film, Ted humors the attendant's insistence on operating the camera. So Ted clowns for the camera, amusing those around him with the manner in which he can suggestively maneuver and deploy his tongue. Tolerant of the storekeeper's absconding with the apparatus, he shows similar consideration in musing upon a shadowy male figure caught briefly walking in the park. This is Richie, son of a long time female acquaintance, who is "mixed up", or so Ted ruminates. He muses on the good some institutionalization might do Richie, if only just to find out "what's wrong".

And so, this film does what Ted thinks it does. It shows us around, but in so doing it remains a very personal perspective, an introduction to his own personality: his concerns over competence, his attention to difference and detail, his worry about figuring even confusing things out, his buffoonery, his generosity. Such traits color his monologues delivered to the smoke filled room; they go with him out into the smoggy city.

"MY OLD MUSIC OF MINE:" ON BEING ALONE

Ted has taped an occasional diary during our research contact. Here, he portrays making it through several days:

Well let's see. Now gettin' up now. It's ten minutes to one (p.m.). Thursday. Hell, I don't know what the hell I'm going to do today. Guess I'll go down here and get some coffee. Go down and get something to eat. Walk around, downtown, and see if there's anything different, and what else. Oh, I'll guess I'll play some of my, some more of my rare old music of mine. My, I love the music of mine. Bing Crosby. Ahhhh, now, let's see.

Friday. I guess I'll go down to the laundiemat (*sic*) and see how everything is down there. Then, see if everything's all right. Then come back, get something to eat. Walk around. Down at the park. Feed my little birds, my little sparrows. Go over there and talk to Tim over in park. Thing's open there. And take a little, oh, walk around and shoot the bull and I'll come back home and have something I can, else to eat in the restaurant. Do a little work around there: wash the dishes, the pots and pans. Then talk to the cook and dishwasher, (tape unclear) with them a little bit. Then I come home, nine o'clock (p.m.). Get ready to go down to Pico at 9:15 (p.m.). Then I go down and do my laundiemat and then I come home. And watch T.V. until five in the morning. And then I took my bath and went to bed and I woke up. *It's Saturday.* Now it's the thirtieth. I get up and wash up, go down and get something to eat. And I guess I'll go down and, the park for a little bit. See if Tim's over there somewhere. Walk around. Take a day off today. I don't work nowhere. I guess I'll watch the ball game. I don't know. It's been so hard to know what I'm doing. Old man! Feel misable (*sic*)! Oh, hell! What the hell I should do now? Oh, guess I'll play some more of my old music. Yeah, I'll get up and play some more of my old music of mine.

The entry is typical of Ted's daily life, patterning the routine nature of it. He includes stopping by Gordon's Restaurant for coffee, a meal, and some companionship with occasional potwashing or messenger duties in exchange for such nurturant amenities. At the time of this diary entry, Ted had a laundromat which he tended with a protective as well as custodial eye. But overall, his mind passes from setting to setting with a transient sense of touching regular points of reference, between which he takes his pleasure with an explorative indulgence in familiar settings, his jazz record collection, or his functional television screen. Striking is his demonstrated ease in the midst of an imposingly risk-laden environment. It is not that he fails however to appreciate or weigh the inconvenience, the personal hassles, or the odds of his surroundings.

Dealing with the wildlife, Ted shows favoritism. On the one hand, he prides himself on the sparrows, "some red, some white, some grey" which indulge in the feed which Ted stocks across his room's windowsills. Ted is particularly fond of one monoped sparrow, and enjoys the persistent chirping of them all as feeding time "once in the morning, once at night," approaches.

With similar benevolence, he welcomes mice which regularly partake of seed fare spilled from the sills.

On the other hand, against the pigeons forever out for more than their share of the hand-out, or the cockroaches prone to venture across his walls, he is a vigilant foe.

Pigeons eat all day and shit all day. Sparrows, they just peck, constantly pecking. Pigeons are as noisy as flies. You can hear their wings flying. Keeps me up half the damn day, just keepin' the pigeons away!

"It blinds 'em for life" he explains of the ammonia he stocks in a needled syringe and a plastic squirt gun, either within reach to be aimed at noisy pigeons. He can swamp a cockroach, a moving target some fifteen feet to a high ceiling corner, from his reclining vigilance atop his bed; at his leisure, he dispatches their writhing forms not far from where they have fallen. Despite the odds, the inventive complexity of his battle affords him certain pleasure.

Against human foes, Ted also maintains a weapon, a club of impressive proportions. He advises me that "the law" states that as long as "they" stay outside his room, he can't touch potential intruders. "But the minute they stick their heads in my window", he is free to dispatch them as he wills. With hand upon his staff, he one night stared with cunning stillness and, he admitted later, a degree of terror as his door knob persistently rotated back and forth, firm in the hands of a potential assailant. Who the victim of the apparently inevitable confrontation actually would have been is not clear from Ted's account of his bed-ridden attendance to the matters at hand. In advance, he had envisioned an intruder swamped by merciless defenses; as the stranger's steps receded from his door, he found himself surprised by the paralytic fear he had experienced.

While residing in a Cherry Street hotel, day and night Ted was alone in defiance of such threats. He reported that thieves, on several occasions when he was absent from this room, "kicked the goddamn door in". On the door, he attempted to devise locks of his own; he complained that he also had to "lock the goddamn windows every goddamn time I go out" despite the fact that he lived on the third floor, albeit near a fire escape.

One guy down here, got his fuckin' brains all beat up! Eyes like this! (Ted emphasized the victim's swollen face with fingers spread before his eyes). They beat the hell out of people out here. The cops have been down here so damn much. Shit, I'm goin' nuts!

Of consequence to Ted, but primarily inconvenient to him, was a murder in the hall just outside his room: his primary complaint was over having to stay in his room after the violence, something ordered by the police, which had him "pissing in the goddamn sink and no coffee or nothin'" for a full twenty-four hours. Finally, he figured he had been an obedient citizen long enough. For weeks thereafter, Ted maneuvered his bulky frame around the imposing blood stain on the hall rug. Ted figures that his best defense is to "mind my own business" and "do nothin'". He believes this approach protects him from the violence and sometimes affords him perquisites, such as his landlord arranging a streetside, third floor room with windows affording Ted a ringside perch over Cherry Street.

But the murder, the predictability of beatings, the break-ins are indeed vexing, if even, in Ted's presentation of them, only inconvenient. And yet, Ted finds an avocation in investing personal effort against the odds. One early morning, Ted deliberately descended to the lobby fire door in order to witness the intention of two suspicious characters he had watched from his room windows. Having attempted to pry the cigarette machine for its cash, the couple exited for a short time; in the interim, Ted slipped into the lobby, removed the as-yet-unpilfered cash, and retreated to his room to harbor the money for his landlord while the would-be thieves hacked away with a retrieved crowbar. Whether in fact the same attentiveness saved the Continental Insurance Tower several years ago, the smoke from which Ted spotted in the early morning hours and claims to have pointed out to the sleeping engine company across the street, depends on with whom one speaks. Ted contends that he alerted the Los Angeles Fire Department about the fire which won them considerable national recognition in the art of battling towering infernos. The engine company commander fails to recall anything about a burly unshorn man ambling to his door, and instead acknowledges his electronic equipment's role in spreading the general alarm.

The hassle of one too many doors kicked-in was a catalyst for Ted, who then moved from Cherry Street to a hotel with a twenty-four hour desk manager. In his new neighborhood, he finds the sparrows as eager, the pigeons as deliberately despoiling, and the insectivore and human "cocka-roachies" as ever present. Still, he misses the pleasure of a fresh cigar on Cherry Street at two-thirty in the morning, taking in the looming, impressive hulk of the insurance tower and savoring the night stillness of the inner city. Things are more crowded in his new location: a brick wall for a view, a canyon of brownstones out front, and since he is nearer the park, more of the bustle of people. Still, he knows his ease in being alone, whether watching out for the spoilers or eventually retreating to his much loved record collection of Benny Goodman and his era.

"I'M NO LOCKED-UP PATIENT": BEING STREET-WISE

Ted's present living arrangements demand from him several adaptive strategies which have emerged over his life's course: (a) a set of hobbies and diversions, (b) a charade of mental illness, (c) bravado and joking buffoonery, (d) an inter-personal reserve, (e) self-reliant independence, (f) an ability to retract from danger, and (g) a benefactor role. These strategies, Ted's adept juggling of them, provide the focus of this next section.

A SET OF DIVERSIONS

Besides the watchfulness he maintains, Ted engages in several considerably less risky enterprises.

I'm no expert on coins, but uh, you see uh, I sic (*sic*) 'em off the liquor store's business 'cause they don't want 'em. I get the two dollar bills from them so they don't have to take 'em to the bank, deposit 'em. So I just do it to save 'em. Save 'em money. That's the only way I can save money. Save two dollar bills. 'Cause nobody, don't like 'em. The liquor stores hate 'em because they ain't got no place to put' em (in the cash register drawers).

In preparing for his bi-yearly visits to see his sister, he notes:

I'm all the time going through coins, I'm going through half dollars. I got this here, I got uh, things to look at when I got nothing to do. I got my dimes I roll up. I got pennies I got rolled up. I got coins to go through. Got to save 'em for my kids. I'm lookin' for new, new half a dollars, new quarters. I take 'em out and put 'em in here, and when I get ten dollars' worth I roll 'em up and I put 'em in the, in the drawer. It's just somethin', I got somethin' to do when it's too damn misable (*sic*), I'm too hot or nothin' good on T.V. to do.

Paying no heed to his sister's warnings about envelopes mailed thick with paper currency, Ted continues to count on the virtue of the U.S. Postal Service by mailing the stacks of bills to her. She is incredulous each time a stash makes it through, and faithfully deposits the money in an account for Ted. As for the coins, Ted's own pockets bear them as semiannual treasure for her children.

Collecting is more than an occasional hobby for Ted; often it is at the core of his day. Several months have been filled with avid taping of his record library on a temperamental tape recorder left with him by his brother. Ted figures that two copies of each recording are better than one. Hospital school records from his fourteenth and fifteenth years note his abilities at recognizing numerals and doing transcriptions. With these skills, but no reading ability, he recognized dates, initial letters to Hollywood stars' names and their movies, and having so consulted his weekly *TV Guide*, designs a week's television viewing curriculum. Once viewed, some films for the fifth or sixth time, movie titles and issue dates are transferred to a catalogue, organized by star names. By his indexed account, his viewing history is impressive although at the mercy of late, and late-late, night television.

BEING "CRAZY"

However adept the order and industry of Ted's recreative sense, it is in his self-presentation on the street, in restaurants which he frequents, at laundromat or liquor store work sites, and while wandering the downtown area that the burden of his formerly institutionally-defined incompetence is most evident.

If you can't read or you can't write and you can't go out and get a job, anywhere, you're retarded! People are afraid to go and ask people for a job and get a job, because you can't read or write, they'll find out. They know they are going to make a sucker out of you. They know that they can get you for nothin' practically. If you can't read or write they know they are gonna get you for as cheap as they can get you for. Because if you don't know how to talk for yourself and ask you want more money, you want more what we are supposed to get, they know you never say nothin'. You're gonna talk or you're not gonna come right out and tell 'em. But my mind, since I came out from the hospital, my mind is not even normal. I just don't have the nerve to ask people, "I want more money." 'Cause I know the answer I will get. They are not gonna pay you a salary if you can't read or write.

For Ted, competence is gauged precisely by the ability to read and write. While he still doesn't "know why they put me" in the mental hospital at fourteen years of age, he is most clear that during this year and half tenure there he "didn't belong" in the hospital school. As a student, he attended to the "same thing over and over and over" and has never forgotten how his inability to retain any of the basic skill training was "like a wall". Subsequently, without acquired literacy skills, Ted could not get "good jobs". Through the 1960s and early 1970s, his more recent work history, he has been obliged to accept the "odd job" which "the average person wouldn't do".

His neighborhood is a "rough place to work", yet it is to his liking that, during late night laundromat or liquor store clean up, "nobody's here when I'm all by myself. I got the keys and everything so I just come in and do my job." In the early seventies, Ted was holding down several such billets: sweeping and ordering Skitch's Liquor Store from five to eleven p.m., thereafter heading on to "the laundiemat on Seventh, Union and Pico" at about two-thirty a.m.; by four to four-thirty a.m., he was cleaning a "Sixth Street laundiemat" and, following a seven a.m. coffee break at a doughnut shop, managing the night's disorder in a bar until noon. "Then, I'd get up at four-thirty (p.m.) and start the same thing all over again. Over and over, seven days a week, every day." Out of all this personal industry, Ted was drawing a barely subsistence income.

While he recognizes the extent of his skills and the limits they impose on job opportunity, he nonetheless finds others' awareness of his limitations integral to his being locked into such a self-destructive employment pattern.

They see me in the park and they see me downtown. They see me walking the streets. Even if I dress-up like a clean man, but they see me. They know what I can do, but they see me. They know what I can do, but they know I can't do nothin' else. They know I can't get a good job. They know I worked in sanitoriums. They know I get two dollars a day.

Thus, if only for the connections such employ had for him during his parolled ten years as a sanitarium custodian in several locations, he continues to be haunted by those he perceives to be spotting him, watching him, planning for him.

It is little wonder therefore that, in 1960 when researchers made contact with him, Ted exclaimed, "Everybody knows me! That's why I been gettin' nowheres the last twenty years!" and feared that the contact presaged another tenure at Pacific State Hospital. Though Ted has never exhibited reluctance at cooperating in research efforts, by 1972 at the second researcher contact, Ted would facetiously curse the "stool pigeon" that had let on to his where-abouts. Thus, while he has admirably coped with the unannounced appear-ance of strangers holding a personal interest in him, what such persons might be after, or what the consequences might be of their inquiries, has weighed upon him.

Nevertheless, Ted's long-standing investment in maintaining ties with even ancillary aspects of a welfare delivery system, including researchers, is instructive. Ted recalls his fourteen and a half years on hospital parole as a functioning member of various communities.

They keep putting another person on me to try and discharge me. And I says, "No, I don't want no discharge!" I says, "I want to stay, I want to stay on probation", 'cause the State knows me better mostly than anybody does. If I get in trouble or the law picks me up, I got all the time, get the State to stick up for me. Because the State knows I never do nothin'.

He sincerely suspects that the States, and of late a group of researchers, know him better than he himself does. As such, they may be an anchor for a self-image which Ted finds troubling, and at the very least problematic to his job security. But beyond this, such links are benefactors on reserve. To State intervention, he attributes recurrent prompt release from charges of loitering made years ago; this was a time when he was not yet recognized by police regulars in Ted's post-parole neighborhood. He knows that researcher concern assisted his application for social security benefits for the handi-capped, and thus liberated him from having to hustle five jobs simultaneously in order to make a living. Such times are tangible to his interest in main-taining his identity as a "crazy" person.[3]

A neighborhood friend, Tim, does not accept Ted's occasional boisterous nature, swaggering mimicry of homosexual effeminate locomotion, or delibe-rate attempts to astonish those unfamiliar with his routines as evidence of a deranged mind. Tim is overtly disparaging of Ted's attribution of such behavior to his "crazy" mind. However, others' similar sentiments do not diminish the persistence of this self-presentation by Ted. More than a device for the amusement of others or the provocation of Tim's impatience (though both give Ted great pleasure), such displays and the accompanying explana-tion are strategies with which Ted approaches his daily life.

Following a theft from his room of his diligently saved and counted two dollar bills and rolled coins, I asked him to consider banking (with tellers' help) as a preventive measure against the consequences of another such break-in. Intransigent to the suggestion, Ted based his resistance on a platform of several objections.

(1)   He had replaced the lock on his door after somebody had entered the room previously with a hotel master key, so "they" should not have made it in this time.

(2)   His sister banked money for him already, so there was no need for another account.

(3)   "Because I'm crazy, and I don't know a damn thing about how to do it, or what to write. I am stupid! I don't know nothing!"

(4)   "They cleaned me out already", so there is no point in starting any banking now.

(5)   He's doing a favor for the liquor stores, so he will continue to horde money in his room anyway.

(6)   Nobody knows he has money in his room.

(7)   If a bank did it all, he would not have "something to do with his spare time", i.e., counting and packaging the money.

Presented in the order with which Ted took exception to my insistence and concern, this protocol is important. For faced with the premise of a record of break-ins against him and near certainty of it continuing in the future, Ted at first makes two specious inferences. Perhaps suspecting his own self-deception, or more likely faced with my incredulity, he lands squarely on the "crazy" tag as an attempt to definitively close the conversation. I stress the role of helpful tellers, and Ted proceeds with three more *non sequiturs* to the obvious facts. Then he opts for the recreative relevance of abundant coin and currency. Having "something to do" in counting and recounting the cash emerges as perhaps the most convincing of the arguments, but it was a long way down Ted's own list.

In any case, Ted would have preferred to stymie this complex social exchange by recourse to an explanation of "craziness". As I have seen him employ it in countless potentially prolonged and imposing conversations, Ted attests openly to the efficacy of a "crazy" image in severing anti-social threatening situations such as he has occasion to meet on the streets or in the cramped hallways of his residency hotels. However, there is an important contrast in the image's use, depending upon the context in which it is utilized. In fending off the human wildlife, Ted summons the strategy with deft control. In answering for his own errors of judgment or confusion over conversational distinctions, it is his feared or overt loss of control which renders a sufficient condition for its use. When I once pressed him to distinguish between an "aunt" and an "uncle", terms used indiscriminantly in one of his narratives to the point that I was confused, he rejoined:

I don't know. One is our uncle. Let's see. I got me in a hole there. I wish I knew what it was. My head is to slipped, there's nothing much to it!

The verbal manipulation of being "crazy" is a useful veneer for Ted's deep concerns over his incompetence: his inability to find good work, to take exception to others' opinions, and to generally get ahead. As a label with attributes of behavioral usefulness, he can shelter his personal welfare with it. But there are limits to the gloss. Walking with my wife and me along the Venice boardwalk one weekend, Ted was astonished by the sights provided by a community featuring the best and the worst of alternative lives. The talented and would-be musicians, the roller skaters scantily clad, the hawkers of crafts and drug related hardware, the weaving drinkers were all anomalous for Ted, but they were otherwise a credible part of the scenery. But the prone mumblings and twisting of an angel-dust user were a sign, as Ted put it, for "check-out time". Ted was not only on a tour of the seaside fringes of a city, but of the recognizable limits between the "crazy" and the out-of-control. He knew the distinction, and knew his place was far afield from even the gray areas in between. Perhaps that margin, and his certainty about it, permits him ready access to a "crazy" presentation strategy. But the clarity of this one behavioral spectrum and his management of it must occasionally highlight for him the confusion over a retardation label and concomitant history which he never chose, and most certainly has never really understood.

Faced with the pressure of a Thematic Apperception Test given him in the early 1970s, he exclaimed, "You know damn well I'm retarded. I wish I wasn't, but that's the way it goes". His sanguine proposals for correctional therapy have always seemed an afterthought; as he put it on this occasion, "maybe some shock treatment would do it". He has always held some hope for a therapeutic egress from a mental "illness". But his later years have found him referring less and less to cures and, while frustrated with his disability, increasingly sure of himself in the perpetuation of a self-management strategy, a remedy to his daily difficulties, over which he is master.

BRAVADO AND JOKING BUFFOONERY

Much of the time, bravado and joking as social intercourse will obviate Ted's need for exhibited "crazy" behavior. Ted enters a medical clinic, for care of an erupted cyst on his back, and a nurse mispronounces his last name.

Ted: Can't even pronounce my name right!
Nurse: Well, how do you want me to say it? (With sarcasm) B—A—R—R ... "Bar", E—T—T ... "ett".
Ted: "Bearit!" "Bearit!"
Nurse: Oh? You ... "Bearit". I don't see no "e" in there!"
Ted: (With disdainful mimicry): "I don't see no 'e' in there!"
N: No, I don't see no B—E—A—R, do you? (Turning to the nurse's aide).
T: Well, it's "Bearit" (Under his breath).
N: That's "Barit!"

T: Learn how to spell. You got it on my card there!; how to spell it.
N: B—A—R—R—E—T—T.
T: "Bearit". You like, go back, go back to where you come from!
          (Smiling).
N: I was born and raised here.
T: Yeah, you better stay here, too!
N: (Laughing): Right here. I'm right where I came from.
T: Yeah, you better stay here too. Yeah. (The nurse suggested we
          wait in the waiting room.) No hurry! You ain't goin' nowhere;
          neither am I.

As is often the case with repartee as one of Ted's presentational strategies, the first to the last word of this conversation centers on the issue of incompetence: first, in the nurse's failings to pronounce Ted's name correctly, and finally in Ted's suggestion that he and she, because of their mutual limitations, were going nowhere with no promising future.

Ted's bullish persistence in such badinage often succeeds, perhaps as much because of his two hundred and twenty pound frame as anything else. In addition to commanding respect from strangers, his massive body turning and swaggering, or playfully feigning coquetry, elicits a humored moment from the most dedicated of teases and long-time friends. Thus, with behavioral hyperbole, even in the most threatening of circumstances, Ted can be overtly very sure of himself. Referring to his perspective on what he claimed to have been police harassment some twenty years before, Ted asserts:

They don't take me to jail because I'm a man! I own this town! I'm fifty years old; I own this town! I don't worry about the police. To hell with them! They didn't stop, be money (*sic*) taken out of my room, did they?

Such bravado usually surfaces with friends, most often in Gordon's Restaurant where such behavior is expected from him. In this setting, Ted is boisterous about his encroaching impotence.

I'm a man all over. Down here (pointing to his genitals), I'm no, no man. But up here I am! This is no good; this has had it. Dead as a door nail.

There is both justification and refuge in such bold proclamations of worth and worthlessness as a man. Friends' disbelief over the veracity of Ted's mental disability may actively inspire Ted to be brazenly open to the companionship such assertions of more tangible abnormality could afford him. But approaching and turning fifty years old has been a major trial for Ted, and overt references to his sexuality are symptomatic of the thought Ted has given to the aging process.

In November of 1976, Ted commented, "I don't know. Your mind getting older. It's getting something; I don't know what it is."

Forty: that's when your trouble starts. When you go, when you get to forty, you're going up a little ways, maybe five, maybe six years, they (sic), you start going down after you get past fifty. Then you start back up again a little bit more, in your late fifties.

I asked Ted to explain why it was that there was an "up" portion to turning just fifty.

Because, when you, you get to forties, then you get the late forties, they, you get the, you go down, then you back up again at fifty; at fifty you go back up again a little bit more; then sixties, that's when you start goin' up, goin' down much further, down where you was at before again.

Ted's image of the aging process resembles that portrayed in Figure 1. The individual rallies with each turn of a personal decade, but ages overall by plunging further faster into the depths.

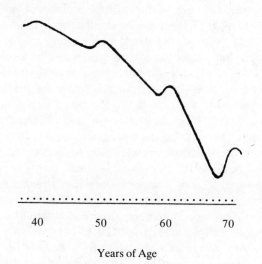

40   50   60   70

Years of Age

Fig. 1. Ted's concept of aging.

(the pitch of the downward movement increases from one personal decade to the next, making the rise at the turn of each decade more difficult for the individual)

It goes right up again, it goes back down again! That's the change of life. You only live so, only so many years. They, when you get a certain age, uh, either your feet goes out or your, or your mind goes out. It could be one of the two. It's usually your feet goes bad; you can't walk good like you used to. Or your mind gets a little bit wor, worse than it was, than it is. 'member, 'member anything, or you don't 'member anything. I remember I was, I was dressing myself, I clothes myself, I know when to eat, I know where to go. But uh, I can't read nothing when I go there and I just have to memorize things.

Ted notes how much harder it is to memorize, to see, and his feet are "gettin' too old to run fast no more. I tried it. I just can't do it no more". And yet, for Ted, the aging process is taking its biggest toll with his sexuality.

Ted's own theory of personality has always been steeped in sexual identity.

Some people are cold, some people are warm, some people are hot. There's nothing to do but, the person that controls himself with sex with a woman. It's natural. Everybody has their own pleasure.

Ted has begun to doubt what he has always taken to be his own "hot" identity; where he once had to "control" his pleasure, he now finds that potential partners, pornographic pictures of both sexes alone or together, and even the suggestive innuendoes from others "don't bother me". Which is to say, they leave him quite unresponsive, quite "cold".

At Pacific State Hospital, despite surgical recommendations to the contrary, Ted refused to sign informed-consent forms for his own sterilization, a procedure which he was sure would make him "weak" and most certainly "cold". But maintaining his identity is no longer a case of summoning a fiercely independent spirit to the cause of resisting hospital administrators. Nor is his emergent impotence something which can be as carefully managed as his "craziness" has been for all these years. Age is providing him with a handicap which he can neither resist outwardly nor control inwardly so as to devise useful strategies to disguise it. On the street as a "crazy" person, Ted has always been able to turn the stigma on and off. And always he could retreat to this room, his catalogues, music, and cigars, to a private world in which mastery of his chosen domains of pleasure was assured.

Now, his handicap does not disassociate itself in his private life. With a direct link established in Ted's mind between a personality concept, upon which he categorizes all people, and his own sexuality, a reduction in sexual prowess is a good deal more encompassing than it would be for most adult males. For a person with a diffused social and occupational history, there is little behind the bravado about the shift in a decade. Ted feels he *is* a different person simply because he *is* fifty years old; a core to his private past, and future, is dissolving. The audience of the Gordon's Restaurant regulars perhaps oblige him the audience for joking declarations asserting the costs of being "crazy" and impotent. At least the former trait is manageable. It makes up for knowing how out of control is the link between age and impotence.

AN INTER-PERSONAL RESERVE

At fifty years, Ted insists that he alone is the "Big Daddy" or "Hot-Dog Man" of Los Angeles gay males, declaring his personal legend to the amusement of those around him. Braggadocio aside however, he is cautiously aware and prides himself that he "can smell a 'queer' in a town like a book of matches". He is indulgent to some who have benign, perhaps prurient, motives relative to him. Ted enjoyed one fellow, years back, who kept returning once a week with his new Polaroid camera and "testing it out" in Ted's room. Each visit, he would apologize for the failure of his apparatus on the previous visit; each time he would promise to get it right so that nude photographs of Ted really would come out. For his generosity, perhaps naiveté, Ted retains but one sprawled shot of his generous bodily form and has, in any case, lost track of the man. Ted once patiently endured the process of having a plastic mold made of his naked body, serving as a clear plastic base for an artisan's apartment lamp. Ted once saw the product of his profile, but he has long since given up keeping track of the artist's domiciles so as to arrange viewings for friends.

Along with such encounters is the occasional homosexual experimentation which life at Pacific State Hospital established as a normative aspect to ward, and generally interpersonal, relationships. He relishes stories of male friends astonished and throttled by his endowments; more typically he clowns endlessly and occasionally flirts with gay friends. But he is aware of the excesses of this sexual domain, often conjuring images of the victimization and consequences of sexual abuse witnessed in his short but traumatic institutional life while a teenager. Thus, on the street, Ted takes pride in instincts he claims identify, beyond the idiosyncratic inter-personal styles of some, the dangerous intentions of others. In any setting, he separates those who will "have 'spect for me" and those who would victimize. Ted routinely accompanies an aging prostitute friend on her weekly expeditions to Public Market in order to allay her fears of assault. On such walks, he pegs for himself, or for a companion, the pick-pockets, "winos", and mentally disturbed who are to be keenly watched and avoided. Bravado, it seems, can only get Ted so far in his world; a good measure of preventive awareness can make an important difference in a marginal, threatening landscape.

SELF-RELIANT INDEPENDENCE

Only three times, in the two years of our regular meetings, did Ted call me on the telephone. As he once put it, "Do what you gotta do with your work! Don't worry about me". Ted continues to assume that should I want to visit him, I will make the effort; conversely, only occasionally and casually has he made the bus journey from the inner city to Venice in order to visit our home. He has never been dedicated to arranging regular meetings or conversations. Such independence has been a coping strategy for Ted over many years.

Before and after his sixteen month hospitalization, Ted reports that he "did odd jobs around the neighborhood. Like yard work. Yea, I did a lot when I was young." Asked how he had found these jobs, he self-sufficiently noted that he "did that on my own. What I find, I find; what I don't find, I don't find." During the late forties and through the late fifties, Ted held several custodial sanitarium jobs, two which he held respectively for two and three year tenures. During his sanitarium employment period,[4] his independent nature asserted itself, sometimes to his disadvantage, even loss of employment. At one sanitarium, he was dismissed for openly complaining to elderly residents about the food as "slop" which neither he nor they should tolerate. But his recurrent disrespect for rules, which he took as unnecessarily harsh or as arbitrarily imposed, developed in spite of reprimands and dismissals.

I said "I go anywhere I want. I'm no locked-up patient. I'm employee (*sic*)." I can go anywhere I want, anytime I want to. Shit, they locked me in; I climbed the goddamn wall and I said, "Hell with you, no way! I'm no locked-up employee here." They got a tall wall that I can climb the son of a bitch. They told me I couldn't do it! I said, "Shit, there's nothin' I can't climb. I'll find a way to get over."

Much of the intensity of this aversion to others' limits seems to have a basis in those months as a young teen-ager at Pacific State Hospital. A good indication of this came after Ted had made the above declaration of independence and Tim had challenged the assertion that Ted could extricate himself from any situation. Tim conjured the image of a locked, padded cell with steel bars and with "nobody openin' the door!" Ted responds:

I'm no locked-up patient. I work there. They hired me to work there! Every sanitarium work I do . . .

Describing an actual situation with which he had coped, vividly evoking a memory from some eighteen to twenty-five years before, Ted employs a descriptive present tense. But Tim insisted that Ted deal with the hypothetical cell where the door would never open, and in which the incarcerated Ted would be fed through a slot in the door.

Ted: How do they give you a bath?
Tim: There's a shower in the cell.
Ted: Hell, they don't!
Tim: Yes, they do. How are you going to get out? Show me!
Ted: I'll find some way to get out. There's no place you can't get out of! I just wait for my time to come. Then I get out.

Tim was still not satisfied, and kept working away at Ted and reminding him that he would be fed to the dogs or shot if he tried to escape, and that the key to his cell would be kept in a very secure place. To such pressure, Ted exclaimed, "They're not going to keep me locked up in no goddamn security!" At this point, Ted's memories were not only being vividly recalled in the present voice, but the conjured cell of Tim's invention had become tangibly oppressive.

I'm a 'ployee! I'm not a patient. I can go anywhere I want to. I'll wait there when they open the goddamn door. They'll open it. I'll tear the goddamn walls down. I seen a crazy guy tear a wall down with his fingers!

The exigencies of institutional and parole life have, by repeatedly frustrating or prematurely severing many of Ted's ties to other people, stimulated further such determined self-reliance. So have Ted's memories of childhood: partial amnesia over the four years following his being hit by an automobile as well as a brief and turbulent two and a half years with his mother and siblings before his admission to the hospital have left little to recall of familial companionship. Even Ted's sister, two years younger than he, speaks but vaguely of fleeting glimpses of home life. The impact that such personal distances can have is clear in Ted's account of missing his father's funeral in 1959.

I used to work on Ninth Street. I work like a dog down there, work twelve hours a day. I put so many hours in, and by the time I got dressed and got my bath, got dressed and got, got to the corner, I already missed the bus! When I got to the uh, sidewalk on Alvarado, I had to wait for another bus. Well, I still can't figure out why it is, why my sister couldn't just uh, drive down here to Third Street, pick me up. 'Stead of me tryin' to catch a bus, 'cause I don't know how the schedule of the bus works.

As a devastating lapse in family relations, this even actuated in Ted a desire to sever contacts with his sister. During the following eleven years, he did not see her, and resumed contact only because a researcher[2] arranged a reunion of all the family siblings. The event and its outcome gives perspective on the risks of Ted's self-reliance.

Of more recent years, Ted observes:

It's a lot of, well uh, it's a lot of questions tryin' to catch buses. That's why I use my bike. I just catch the, use my bike and go where I want to go. I don't have to wait for a bus everyplace I have to go. Get my bike and I go; right now. I don't have to uh, you know, make a certain schedule on a bus stop or I miss the bus or something. That's my problem, see. That's why I have, uh, odd jobs where no certain time. I have a certain time to do it in. Boss don't say nothin'. He knows I do my job. That's all he cares about.

Between Ted's recognition of his own limitations and the potentially abrasive nature of others' expectations, he maintains a free-lancing interface and thus avoids having to cope with the scheduling rules of a normative urban life style. The flexible nature of Ted's personal and work life could integrate, but not need to synchronize with, the routine and regular bus service of the inner-city. And Ted does avail himself occasionally of the bus service. But it is the idea of missing a bus or having to ask "a lot of questions" which is perplexing. Independence of schedules and rules affords a continuation of previously demonstrated, and perceived, competence.

But while evasion *ex post facto* may be the response to having failed to measure up, Ted can readily face complex situations in which failure is highly possible. For instance, on a piece of folded notebook paper which I retrieved from the detritus of Ted's floor, a jumble of numerals seemed purposeful. Ted explained that he had been "figuring" what the hotel manager owed him, after the manager had made a recent deduction from Ted's monthly Supplementary Security Income (S.S.I) check routinely cashed by the hotel. Ted had expected a benefit increase for some two months, and finally, instead of simply endorsing the check as usual when it was presented to him by the manager, he perused the face amount. Agreeing immediately that Ted should receive more, the manager handed over another ten dollars above the usually-expected balance of two hundred and ten dollars. Not convinced that this sufficed, Ted queried once again, and was reluctantly given another three dollars. Even with the thirteen extra dollars, Ted decided to figure the balance himself. Ted's strategy in working out this problem (see Table I)[5] and Ted's own worksheet (Figure 2) indicate the complexity of the task as Ted foresaw and dealt with it.

Ted's first strategy, a breakdown of his check total into units of ten, could have told him all he needed to know. But he could not spontaneously determine the amount due, for his financial map included a set of disparate remainders once he had marked off his seventy-five dollar rent deduction: (1) two tens at the bottom of his numerical column remaining after Ted's demarcation of new one hundred dollar points (see Table I, Step 3), (2) a five left from the ten he had divided to calculate the seventy-five dollar point at which his rent stopped and his spending money would begin, and finally (3) an eight, to total the increased SSI benefits sum of three hundred and eight dollars. To recover all these remainders was not an easy process of scanning and adding.

So, beginning some long, hard work with three more methods for determining his due, he gets very close to having the exact amount, after rent deduction, when he makes a large addition error. A mistake in carrying (Table I, step 7) does him in here. Realizing something is amiss, Ted turns to subtraction as a third strategy, but fails to perform any operations with it. The figures, set three times on the page, do not calculate for him. So, returning to addition as a fourth approach, he decides to (a) find out what in fact he had received, before (b) trying to calculate what he should be getting. Returning to the breakdown, he apparently finds the unconsidered remainders, and subsequent to accurately adding up the sum of three hundred, locates the eight and reaches the sum of three hundred and eight dollars. He checks his work twice, juxtaposing the numbers, and then compares the total he had been reluctantly handed by the manager with this sum. An error in this last operation indicates he still did not confirm a discrepancy of ten dollars which remained due him.

In talking about the worksheet, Ted was cursory in his attentions. Appearing essentially uninterested, he indicated that he still did not know what was owed him in the months ahead. He persistently minimized his concerns over

TABLE I

Ted figures his monthly due

Decision	Operation	Outcome
(1) Breakdown the new S.S.I. check total ($308.00) into units of ten (abacus style)	Writes a column of tens to equal 300, and inscribes an "8"	Success
(2) Deduct rent total ($75.00) from this breakdown	Counts seven tens and five from the top of column breakdown	Success, but puts remainder "5" (from split of eighth ten) in wrong column
(3) Determine remaining dollars	Marks off new $100 intervals, beginning with marked "75" "Arrows" distinguish these demarcations from previous ones	Possible error in marking last $100 may have led to $210 as the remainder. (this was total received in cash previous to increase in benefits, once rent had been deducted) Should be $220, plus $8.00 which Ted also fails to count
(4) Check to see if abacus total of $210 and rent of $75 equal new S.S.I. total of $308	Addition: $\begin{array}{r} 75 \\ 210 \\ \hline 285 \end{array}$ 308	Success in operation, but writes "308" since 285 = 308
(5) Check work done in (4) by reversing order of numerals	Addition: $\begin{array}{r} 210 \\ 75 \\ \hline 285 \end{array}$	Success in operation, but total does not equal 308; checks breakdown of tens and finds "missing" ten excluded by first perusal
(6) Check to see if $220 and $75 equal the S.S.I. total	Addition: $\begin{array}{r} 220 \\ 75 \\ \hline 295 \end{array}$	Success in operation, but total does not equal 308; checks breakdown of tens and finds "missing" five excluded by first and second perusals (remainder of division of eighth ten to deduct rent)

Table I (continued)

Decision	Operation	Outcome

(7) Check to see if $225 and $75 equal the S.S.I. total	Addition: 225
	    75
	  390
		Error: caused by carrying 1 from addition of 5 plus 5 to the one hundreds column (see original). Because of this error, Ted goes on to next approach, the use of subtraction. Had the addition been accurate, Ted might have solved the problem here, since he would have located, perhaps, the as yet unconsidered "8"

(8) Without using "abacus", determine cash due after $75 deduction by manager	Subtraction: 308 75	Operation not performed
(9) Ditto of (8)	Subtraction: 308 75	Operation not performed
(10) Consider another method of determining cash due	Writes figures involved	
(11) Determine cash due by deducting previously received allowance from present total	Subtraction: 308 210	Operation not performed: Was this due to (a) Ted recognizing that he could not perform the operation, or (b) Ted recognizing that this failed to include the 75 which would have to be deducted from the 308?

(12) Returning to addition, find total received for a month, including the extra cash paid Ted by the manager when latter realized his "error" of dispensing funds.	Addition: 210
	    75
	    13
	  298
		Success, but does not total 308

Table I (continued)

Decision	Operation	Outcome
(13) Check work done in (12)	Addition: 210 / 75 / 13 / 298	Success, but does not equal 308; checks abacus accounting, finding the previously unconsidered ten and five (see [5] and [6] above
(14) Determine total which should be received for a month, now that "ten" and "five" are added instead of $13 handed by manager to Ted	Addition: 210 / 75 / 15 / 290	Error: Carries 1 to hundreds column instead of tens column (see [7]; perhaps realizes sum including "15" could not be smaller than sum including "13" as in (13)
(15) Check work done in (14)	Addition: 210 / 75 / 15 / 300	Success, but still not equal to 308 having arrived at "300" for the first time, is perhaps cued of forgotten "8" in abacus breakdown
(16) Determine cash supplement due Ted now that check is larger	Addition: (on fingers?) or in upper right hand corner of work sheet	Success (equals 23)
(17) Check to see if addition of 23 to previous numerals gives 308	Addition: 210 / 75 / 23 / 308	Success
(18) (19) Check work done in (17)	Addition: (reverses order of numerals) 75 / 210 / 23 / 308 210 / 23 / 75 / 308	Success

Table I (continued)

Decision	Operation	Outcome
(20) Determine total cash received from manager (after $75 rent deduction)	Addition: 100 210 13 323 223	Error: included a "100" which apparently had been previously inscribed on the paper; realizes error and rewrites "223"
(21) Compare (20) with what Ted should be receiving from now on (after $75 rent deduction)	Addition: 210 23 (sic) 223	Error: first writes "13" and then changes it to "23", still making addition error

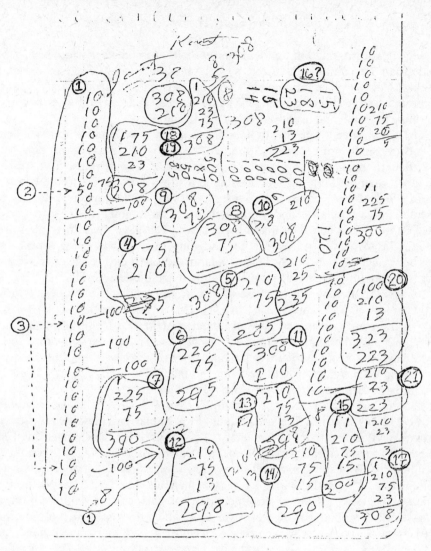

Fig. 2. Ted's worksheet.

the manager's probable routine theft in the past or future. He continued to suspect that he was entitled to more, chose to remain satisfied that at least thirteen dollars had been handed to him in supplement, and resigned himself to his decision not to make a row about any of this. Ironically, after so much hard effort, a final error kept him from the discrepancy he knew he deserved; he had tried himself to figure it out. Failing that, the most he would enigmatically editorialize about the event, he scrawled across the top of his worksheet: a firmly self-deprecatory, "I *can't* kount (*sic*)".

EVASION OR BACKING-OFF FROM DANGER

In such landlord relations and in his verbally combative custodianship of
laudromats frequently vandalized by neighborhood youths, Ted recognized
the limits of his observational skill and his two hundred and twenty pound
frame in meeting direct challenged. Under stress, Ted can and does become
unwilling to go beyond usually effective posturing.

Ted has survived hold-ups in liquor stores, but it was the increase in their
frequency, and more deadly armaments employed, which gave him the
incentive to back out of night-time liquor store stewardships. Two pistol
equipped men held him up one evening in a store. With access to the burglar
alarm blocked by the intruders' entry positions, Ted summoned his most
threatening countenance and warned them, "You're going to have to make
the first move!" When they made their move, Ted gave them their pleasure
without resistance. In retrospect, the indignity of it all was being found the
next morning, tied up on the floor, behind the open cash register, with the
store cat contentedly curled up on his cramped and hindered body.

In less threatening circumstances, Ted's approach is "if it doesn't look
good or feel good to me, I just leave it". His current immobilization in the
face of a recently diagnosed case of diabetes, stemming from the inconvenience he finds attending carefully to his high-sugar and carbohydrate diet,
could have serious consequences for him. But in most cases, this conservative
strategy affords steady ground; without too many decisions, one avoids error
and perhaps confronting recurrent examples of incompetence.

Ted enthusiastically raves, for example, over Tim's living arrangements in
subsidized city housing. Ted could qualify for similar facilities; Tim has been
strong-willed in his desire to facilitate the paperwork for the change. But Ted
does not pursue what partly seems a straight fiscal issue: with cooking
facilities in subsidized housing, Ted would forfeit thirty dollars per month in
SSI payments from the State. Less cash in hand, for Ted, is a persuasive
argument against anything. Another part of this reserve is based on a
long-standing repugnance he feels over food which he has smelled during the
cooking process, a visceral response developed and maintained since his
years working with sanitarium kitchens. But most significantly, Ted does not
want to lose free access to the park neighborhood. He would be somewhat
removed from the enclave, and have to bus over to it were he to move. But
he is also apprehensive over the possibility of "nobody coming up to see"
him in his apartment. He abhors the idea of a doorman who could "stop
them come up (sic) to see me", standing in the way of the park people with
whom he would want to pass the time.

Ted has also been intransigent to the idea of moving to the California high
desert where, on his sister's horse farm, he would have room and board and
a paying job as a ranch hand. It's a beautiful spot, by his own admission and
although the work is unfamiliar, he has little doubt that he could soon

August, John Hopper, a black man appearing to be in his mid-thirties (though actually 42) moved into the apartment. Penny, who had met him at the beach, was caught once again in a flurry of plans for marriage, a trip back East to visit John's family and the possibility of moving from the apartment to a house so that they could get a dog. She referred to his car as "their car" (though he was quick to correct her) and began subsidizing its rehabilitation. John worked only infrequently and for little money and spent a fair share of his time entertaining himself outside of Penny's company, but he often drove her places and was generally kind.

By December 1981, Penny and John were still together but unmarried; even if the major character in Penny's life had changed, the script remained basically the same. As calm and unconcerned as ever, she continued to live the life she had arranged for herself, inured to and seemingly unaffected by its constant flux, unbothered, ostensibly, by its tenuous security; untroubled by the future; and unaware, apparently, that hers was a life upon which melodramas are modeled.

DISCUSSION

What becomes clear in looking at Penny's life history is that radical changes took place in her support system over the course of her life, resulting in equally radical changes in her life circumstances. For the first 33 years of her life, her parents were the focal members of her support network. Admittedly, not all of those years were ideal. Nevertheless, Penny's parents kept her clothed, fed, and reasonably presentable. They guaranteed her inclusion in an extended family network, the benefits of which included warmth and acceptance, a place at the table on holidays and other family gatherings, presents on her birthday and Christmas, and so forth. They served as insurance that she would remain in the home in which she had grown up and in the neighborhood she knew so well. And above all, they lent her life stability.

These guarantees disappeared, however, when Penny's father died. While Penny's life did not immediately change in any dramatic fashion, his absence increasingly altered the substance of her life as time passed: she found herself living alone; she was left unprotected from those who would victimize her (even if at her own invitation); she was unable to sustain the affective ties which had previously bound her to her relatives; she eventually had her house and neighborhood taken from her; and ultimately entered a very different social milieu characterized by far more transient relationships. In the end, she had travelled from a secure middle-class existence to a far more uncertain life style more closely resembling that of a low-income street person.

Who stepped in to fill the gap left by her father's death? To start, there were Penny's relatives. Whatever their original intentions, the way in which independently. Within a short period of time she had made the acquaintance of any number of individuals in her neighborhood, adding them to an already impressive roster of associates. Some of the old faithful remained: Karen, Mrs. Pelham (until she left town to join her daughter in Colorado without informing Penny of her departure), her cousin at the bicycle shop (whom she invariably dropped in on to borrow money), and the two field researchers with whom she was then involved. But just as noteworthy were the countless acquaintances she would happen upon wherever she traveled. Walking out her door, Penny might encounter Jeremy and Amy, whose one year old was quite often entrusted to her care and who often lent her small amounts of money; Matthew, a neighbor who helped her break into her apartment when she locked herself out and who kept her informed on who had dropped by to see her in her absence; Rick, another neighbor with whom she often exchanged pleasantries; an older woman a few doors down who often gave Penny money for a meal. Walking down the street she might hail the woman who saved newspapers for her so that she could redeem them at the recycling center. Passing the post office she might greet a mailman in a truck with a "hi partner" and shoot off a "Hi Rob" to a mailman who would studiously ignore her, explaining, "He's one of my buddies". Entering the local donut shop, Penny might turn to the man behind her and ask if his dog had returned home yet, noting that he'd had a tumor and had to have surgery. Minutes later she might call all over to a man and teasingly berate him for not being at work, identifying him as a pest control worker. Walking into a restaurant in which she hadn't eaten for years, she could greet the shortorder cook by name, share hellos with the hostess, waitress and bus boy, and finally with-stand the hugs and kisses of the owner. At the pier, she might catch up with Gary, an old school mate who would take her out on his boat, or Stan, a bus driver who sometimes loaned her money. Returning home, she might stop to chat with the florist in the shop by her apartment and shoot the breeze with Ricky, a gas station attendant and McDonald's employee, asking after his car and children. Wherever she went, Penny knew someone; wherever she went, she missed no opportunity to meet someone new.

By June, 1981, J. J. was only erratically appearing at Penny's apartment. She explained that he and a bunch of other men had been in front of a liquor store in the downtown area when a man with whom he was exchanging words slapped him. J. J. stabbed him three times. Unfortunately, witnesses had informed the police that he lived on Penny's street and he was thus reportedly laying low, staying with a friend. (The field researcher suspected strongly that J. J. had concocted this story as a way of diplomatically terminating the relationship.) By July, Penny acknowledged that the relation-ship was over but had little to say about J. J.'s departure. She claimed that he wanted to get back together again but that she had felt it was time for them to separate and was not interested in a reconciliation.

Within a relatively short time, Penny found a replacement for J. J. In victimization at her hands. As he describes it, she calls him in pursuit of his sexual endowments, those of which he was once both proud and generous. With a well-paying customer upstairs in the hotel, Judy is in the habit of calling at Ted's room and, if he is out, leaving at least a glamorous red lips print on his door. Tim is convinced that money motivates her interest in Ted. At the bargain five dollars she expects from Ted for sessions lasting from an hour to an hour and a half, what is had in Ted's company does not seem to be profit. Ted talks with disgust of the twenty-odd cats with which Judy lives, imputing to her the questionable qualities of anyone so inclined. Yet it is with her that he persists in his preoccupation at achieving youthfully frequent sexual pleasure. Judy's physical therapy, along with the offerings of store-front healers and street pharmaceutical hustlers, are the warp and woof of Ted's pursuit of the miracle cure for reduced sexual responsiveness.

Now, along with his calendar-record of Los Angeles Dodgers wins and losses (but no scores), Judy inscribes notice of those occasions upon which Ted, in spite of his memories to the contrary, does indeed recover his sought-after sexual identity.

Ted's relationship with Valerie Carlin, and her son Richard, has lasted nearly twenty years. He was working at a bar when he met her, just before the time Edgerton (1967) first established contact with him.

We started talkin', you know. She already had a girl already. I had to come down and get her one damn day; baby sitter was drunk and the police got her baby. They got her; lost her job. I had to go get her at the police station. She had a girl; a beautiful girl. But she had to give it away. 'Cause she had Richie. She got pregnant again.

Thus, when Ted met her, "she already had Richie in her body yet".

I been taking care of him all this time. Hell, he's almost as big as I am already. I don't make much money, and she's pretty good knowing how to spend money. She knows I don't make much money, so, uh, she knows, how to spend it, what to buy, you know. So I got a little money left myself, buy clothes, get a bike.

Valerie will never be able to pay Ted back for all the money he has lent her and her son, and this in no way concerns Ted. Perhaps as recompense, she does his laundry for him occasionally, and provides, in her apartment, a comfortable retreat from time to time. Probably most significant for Ted is the frank admiration Valerie has for him. Among her prolific (according to Ted) output of poetry, she includes a strikingly original, sensitive, but not overly sentimental description of this friend of hers. She speaks of a potential which never was, but of an identity forged by choice far from the established constraints of an achievement- and accomplishment-oriented world.

Such feelings arise out of a relationship which is familial in nature. Certainly, the tie contrasts with the carnal side of Ted's liaison with Judy, or with the lonely, sometimes drug dependent, usually unhappy professional women for whom Ted has had a fondness over the years. Speaking of his own dismay at Richie's troubles with the law, and the tensions of maternal-offspring relations, Ted sounds much like the bewildered parent.

Aww, he thinks he's a big wheel now. Got one of these like a police call radio, makin' that "Decoy one five 'A', one five 'A', call one two one". His mother asks him to do something and he, "Later, later, later". Supposed to keep the goddamn place clean so that, so they, the other two guys don't say nothin'. But goddamn, why the hell should I do it, go over there and do it, hell. "Have 'spect for your mother, Richie. God, your mother's gettin' old, for Christ's sake. Have to, have to 'spect for her." Christ sake, woman's gettin' up her age. Shoot, he just take, takes money out of her like a, like a fruit cake!

Or later, he describes his role in the home when he is with Valerie and Richie.

He talks back to her, and tells her where to go, what to do, where to go. (Question: How do you get along with Richie?) Me? I'm just like anybody else. I just, he ignores me. She knows it's my fault. I know too, but uh, I just don't say nothin', I don't uh, spank him or nothin'. He does that, he talks back to the mother or something, I don't say nothin'. I just uh, let go, like to sit back to the cigar in my mouth, and quiet, don't say a word. She keeps yellin' at him, keep yellin' at him to do something, and you know, it's uh . . . I'm not going to tell. I've very quiet. I don't say, I don't say much. I just do what I want. I go where I want, and uh, that's it. Uh, I don't go dancin'.

This is a striking reference Ted makes at the conclusion to this monologue. Over forty years before this recollection of Ted's own "parental" failings, it was his father's evenings out with other women, getting a reputation as quite a ballroom "dancer", which began to erode the Barrett marital and family bonds. As the uncontrollable child of social worker reports and the crux of his mother's crisis of control in her domestic life, Ted unconsciously listens as his mother "keeps yellin'". As the father this time around, Ted won't "go dancin'", but he won't be held responsible for how Richie, Valerie's problem child of the present and Ted's projection of himself in the past, finally turns out. In maintaining his membership in Valerie's household for so many years, on a casual visitation basis only, with his own apartment and neighborhood routine and her "other two guys" contributing to the asexual nature of the bond, Ted preserves an unconscious connection with his past. The concern Ted feels about Richie's problems is real, but the fact that Ted does not actively intervene or make overt suggestions to Richie about ways of changing speaks of the primary lessons of Ted's own life: there is little that one can control. A hospital might help Richie to "straighten out". But Ted has never seemed really convinced of that. Perhaps his own experience reinforces that ambivalence. At the very least, he retains something from a parental model: unlike his father, he is not going to abandon those who depend upon him, for whom he holds the role of benefactor.

On the basis of a previously mentioned TAT given to him and interpreted by a clinician at the UCLA Neuropsychiatric Institute, Ted was described as isolated, with a history of arid family relationships, and harboring feelings of inadequacy. He is portrayed as being immobilized in solving problems, and as responding to stress in a relationship by backing off. He is thought to assume that withdrawal and active avoidance of dissension will make discordance disappear. Hostility is seen to be fighting within him. He is not a verbal problem-solver. He cooperates with authorities but characteristically exhibits a "macho" sensibility in doing so. He favors safe ground through indecisiveness.

These results, in the words employed by the TAT report, provide a useful perspective on Ted's strategies for competence in his daily life. While the TAT may have elicited important themes, the clinician's report portrays a personality landscape of traits which is diagnostically forbidding for an adult male in American society. And yet, these same traits, in the context of Ted's inner city life, portray a remarkably healthy, functionally coping individuality. While isolated from family and profound friendships, Ted is privately active in exploring and interacting with the community of which he is a member; by necessity as well as by choice, he is often engaged in recreative resistance to the natural and human odds surrounding him. His manipulation of a charade of mental illness is more than a veneer to shelter apprehensions over inadequacy or incompetence, although elements of such are no doubt there. He finds in the charade a tool not only for protection against undesirable incursion into his personal domain, but a means to retain supportive attention, albeit humored ridicule, from friends. He backs off at times to evade matters of skill competence, but is not averse to mounting a very considerable private effort to figure some things out that bear directly upon him. In response to ambiguity, authority, or superior odds, he may indeed resign himself or defer, but often in socially constructive patterns of joking, repartee, or buffoonery. As a benefactor, he cedes of himself that which will just meet the needs of select others. At times, Ted is indeed hostile toward the judge who, sitting atop his court bench, is the unconscious metaphor of a system which never gave him the opportunity to say outright how wrong was his relegation to a classification as "feeble-minded", the basis upon which he was sent on his way to institutional therapy. In verbally replaying the sexual and power politics of the wards in which he spent but a year and a half of his fifty years, he provides for himself an explanation for the friendships and social patterns in inner city life. His safe ground in the midst of a very risky and complex environment is the conservatism which keeps him out of the country and within the mainstream of the park and its perimeters. In short, as Ted once put it, knowing "how to walk" in the city, with legs spread apart in an ambling gate postured to lower one's center of gravity, is part of making it in his world.

TED AND SOME PARADIGMS FOR INDIVIDUAL GROWTH

That Ted has been able to assemble the kind of repertoire for adaptive behavior which is here reviewed is quite an achievement, particularly if one takes a quick overview of his developmental years. To do this, it is helpful to juxtapose some of Ted's turning points and passages, as he has described them or cited them, with several biological, psychological, and sociological paradigms for individual growth. Table II diagrammatically compares Ted's history and such models for growth.

As the Great Depression leaves the Barrett family resources strained, a first-born child, Ted, is dragged beneath a recklessly driven automobile and nearly killed. Thereafter, when Ted is recovering from the accident, which for Ted looms as the vortex to the problems he includes in his adult self-presentation, the boy's memory fades. His mother begins to suspect disability even though physiologically this is unsubstantiated. In school, Ted falls behind and a first I.Q. test at nearly seven years puts him well within a disabled category. Meanwhile, Ted recalls his father's evenings away from his wife. His mother loses control of her children and openly declares her exasperation with Ted's behavior. Just as Ted's amnesia lifts from this period, his parents separate and the Barrett children are parcelled out among relatives. By any paradigm of normative development, such trauma, instability, and transience at an early age are distinct liabilities.

At puberty onset, when social skill development (Linden and Dourtney, 1953) and identity management (Erikson, 1959) are imposing for the individual, Ted is spending a lot of idle time on the street and is expected by his mother to take considerable responsibility for his own well-being. Ferrying support payments back and forth between his divorced father and mother, Ted is no doubt aware of the instability afforded him by either parent. Having previously disregarded clinical recommendations for the institutionalization of her oldest son, it is just at the time when Ted's mother would have found out about her fifth pregnancy (there had been a still birth) that she applies to Pacific State Hospital for his placement. Lack of space precludes immediate acceptance there, and so Ted was no doubt increasingly aware of the concurrent timing of these developments as his mother grew more visibly pregnant.

When he is accepted, in his early adolescence, when he should have been assuming a more defined sex role, he is integrated into a peer group and kind of sub-culture which is prohibited the overt romantic involvement it seeks. Nevertheless, within the institution, deviant sexuality abounds amongst patients, and it indelibly imprints itself on the mind of this young man. Due to the benevolence of an aunt and uncle, Ted does find himself sharing an "initial work period" (Miller and Form, 1951) with perhaps much of the population around, but within his neighborhood the pressure of youths not so directed shifts Ted's interest away from his work. When most are leaving the family (Levinson *et al.*, 1974), Ted finds himself being rejected by the military while an illiterate friend is nonetheless accepted. He ends up back with his family.

At the "apex of having one's own way" (Cain, 1964), Ted discovers his

TABLE II

Paradigms for individual growth

Biological "Timetable"

Cain, 1964

|<———————————— infancy and childhood ————————————>| |<—— adolescence ——>| |<—— reproductive period

puberty   sexual maturation   maximally effective physique

Psychological "Timetables"

Jung, 1931

|<——— dependence on parents; "chaotic/anarchic state" ———>| |<————————————————————— youth

|<——————— attention to self as a "sin" ——————>|

Cain, 1964

|<———— social experience of child/parent ————>| |<———— apex of "having one's own way" ———————>)
(value formation, responsibility assignation, status ascription)   (Benedict's "Arc of Life")

Buhler, 1935

|<—— need satisfaction ——>| |<—— adaptive self-limitation ——>| |<———— creative expansion

Linden and Dourtney, 1953

|<— Periods of Life: Infancy ——> evolescence ———— latency ———— puberty ———— adolescence —— early adult

Stages of Maturation: instinct supremacy   education of the instincts   Instinct supremacy/social learning   mating-reproductive
pairing |<— peak potential of sensory perception, motor
and retention, intelligence

Erikson, 1959

|<(infancy)>| |<(early)>| |<— play age —>| |<— school age —>| |<————— adolescence —————>| |<————— young adult
childhood

trust   autonomy   initiative   industry   identity   intimacy
vs   vs   vs   vs   vs   vs
mistrust shame,doubt guilt   inferiority   identity diffusion isolation

Sociological Factors

Levinson et al., 1974

Male adult developmental periods: |<— "LF": leaving the family
|<— "GIAW": getting into adult
(fashion initial life structure/
————————)|

Miller et al., 1951

|<— Career patterns: preparatory period (household chores) ——>| |<— initial work —>| |< trial work period
"Great Depression" ———>| |<— World War II —>|

Thematic Periods In Ted's Life

|<———— The Accident Years ————>| |<——— Family Years In Bell ———>| |<——— The Hospital and First ———>| |<— Sanitarium Work Years
Gardens   Employment

Critical Incidents In Ted's Life

1928 1930   1940   1950
|A |o • | |A | | A | A   A | 20   A   25   A |
                    |5 years   10/   child   admission parole- rejected mother to Hillcrest Healthwin
birth birth of hit by birth of concert memories pick-up to Pacific by   dies   sanitarium   sanitarium
4/15   sister auto   brother parents up of -hearing in military working in
death of   separate support court   cabinet
sibling   payments birth of   shop
                                        from father brother
|<— Ted's amnesia —>|

Table II (continued)

contribution to the nurturance of young ------->]

------->][<------- middle age -------->

------- cultural bearing of second half of life – reversal of sex ------->
characteristics; serious attention to self

------->][<------- establishing internal order -------

------- senescence

family creative   social creative   middle adult-------   involution – instinct supremacy ------->
dimensions of human activity

control, learning->][<-------   culmination of involvement in responsible assignments ------->

------->][<-------   adulthood   mature age ------->

generativity   integrity
vs   vs
self-absorption   disgust, despair

world------->]   [<-SD": Settling down->]

dream)   [<------- transition ------->]   (order vs making it)   [<-"BOOM": Becoming one's own man->][<-(mid-life transition)->][<-------restabilization: new life structure-------

------->][<-------   stable work period -------

------- Liquor Store/Laundromat Work Years ------->][<-Five Job->][<------ Welfare Years ------>
Hustle

|<- |30   1960 |<- |<- | 35   40   1970   45   50
jaundice /official
discharge   father   -contact with Edgerton   laundromat and   -contact with   -contact with
dies   -working in bar   liquor store   Gordon   author
fired from   -friendship with Valerie and Richie   work   -several jobs in laundromats,
San Marino   liquor stores

mother dead in a small hotel room after a long bout with alcoholism; begins his career in sanitarium work at the Sunrise. This insulary placement by the Department of Mental Hygiene acts as a kind of home for Ted, and his lengthy tenure indicates his satisfaction with it. But his opportunities there could hardly be considered representative of Benedict's peaking "arc of life" (Cain, 1964). While others are "getting into the adult world" (Levinson et al., 1974) and exploiting their peak potential for learning and retention, motor control, and sensory perception (Linden and Dourtney, 1953), Ted is being governed by institutionally inspired rules which he finds personally excessive. At a presumed peak of creative expansion (Buhler, 1935), Ted is actively negotiating with the Department of Mental Hygiene to maintain his dependence by prolonging his parole. When other individuals are being "family creative" (Linden and Dourtney, 1953) and "settling down" (Erikson, 1959) has begun, Ted is being officially discharged from the friendship and support system of the department of Mental Hygiene. He is excluded from his father's funeral by virtue of his limited familiarity with the urban bus system and conspicuous absence from family plans.

Finally, while senescence brings for most people a period of culminating involvement in responsible assignments and stable work roles (Linden and Dourtney, 1953), Ted barely holds down various liquor store and laundromat jobs. Certainly there is an order, albeit a scattered one, to this period in Ted's life. But there is little of the established stability and support which for most adults is normative and very probably crucial. Ted has few extra-familial contacts with peer groups, few significant family relations, and no membership in the community, school, or professional organizations in which commitment reinforces and legitimizes adult roles in the community context.

Ted's history is a series of incidents and passages out of synchrony with the mainstream life course of his peers as designated by numerous theoretical approaches to life history and development.[6] This fact has to temper our interpretation of whatever organic etiology of Ted's disability which he or others may invoke. At the very least, Ted's history is fertile ground for a developmental interpretation of socio-cultural retardation. Two incidents in particular, a tragic accident and an apparently desperate decision on the part of a disillusioned and increasingly beleaguered mother, have had enduring and all-encompassing consequences for Ted. Ted's own resourcefulness in response to these turnings has been a series of passages during which a finely balanced repertoire of adaptive strategies has emerged.

CONCLUSION

The life history of someone such as Theodore Barrett is not be be measured as a span of time, but as he himself would peruse it. What is needed is a life account which is neither a pure history, implying a chronology fixed or measured on paper, nor a simple personality profile, failing to demonstrate the immediacy of the past's sweep as it imposes upon Ted. So profound have been some of the incidents and passages of Ted's past that he transcibes them from memory to the present precisely as they were experienced or perceived in their temporal reality. In a frequent juxtaposition of the past and present tenses, Ted constructs a social reality of events which to an outsider may seem jumbled, confusing, contradictory, and sometimes irrelevant. But it is this assemblage of purely qualitative experience from the past and present which portrays Ted as he is, and as he continues to live his history from day to day.

Anthropology has gone a long way in reducing the number of sweeping generalizations about the multifarious and multitudinous states of cultural humankind. It often seems that clinicians, theoreticians, social workers, and families think of the minds of the retarded in much the same way that early anthropologists thought of the minds and adaptations of other cultures (Langness, 1982). Since that early work, we are justifiably incredulous over assertions that the range of personality and ability of individuals in third world cultures is somehow less than that which we accept to be true of those living in industrial, technological societies. It is through making the lives of the retarded accessible in life history form that such analogous notions about the disabled will be called to question. Certainly there is a common sharing of experiences among the retarded, even as there is among members of a generation (Cain, 1964). But it is our job to make clear, as Hart (1954) did for Turimpi's sons in New Guinea, that the retarded differ not necessarily in what they have done, but most certainly in how they have done it.

ACKNOWLEDGEMENT

As a member of Robert B. Edgerton's *Cloak of Competence* study (1967), Theodore V. Barrett worked with that social scientist and his associate in the early 1960s. In a follow-up study in the early 1970s, Mr. Barrett spent several months in association with a student researcher, Gordon Creed. The untimely death of Mr. Creed, in the midst of collecting records of his close relationship with Mr. Barrett, left behind but the promise of what his video-taping, recording tape, and preliminary written thoughts would have produced. The present writer wishes to note therefore the generosity of Don Sutherland and other of Mr. Creed's friends and associates in sharing their reflections on Gordon's time with Ted. The author has had the privilege of continued acquaintance with Mr. Barrett and has worked intensely with him for a two year period. Much of the data discussed here has emerged over this latter span of time, but I wish to express my gratitude for the perspectives and contributions of these previous researchers.

NOTES

1. All names of specific locations have been changed, as have the names of all individuals with the exception of Mr. Barrett. The latter exception is made out of respect for an identity which he insists is his own and not that of a pseudonymed other. Ted has no reading skills in a largely literate society, and therefore has no access to the documented history which for most Americans is the framework of self-image. The use of another name would be to take identity as Ted literally lives it and to deny him the history he has so

generously shared with me. It is his sentiment, and my wish, that this remain his life account.
2. Gordon Creed; see acknowledgement.
3. Edgerton and others have suggested that being "crazy" may be a more manageable stigma for individuals labelled "mentally retarded", at least insofar as they meet social demands on their performance. It is important, in this regard, that Ted will rarely use the term "retardation" as an explanation or description to me of his difficulties, and will do so only occasionally in a clinical setting.
4. An abbreviated time line of major aspects to Ted's life is provided by Table II on pp. 185–186.
5. Table I maps out Ted's figuring in terms of decisions, operations performed, and outcomes achieved. These are placed in sequence on the basis of the figures' obvious progressions and each operation's location, and likely order of inscription, on the work sheet. However, the analysis relies to some extent on guess work. Thus, some operations as Ted actually performed them may be slightly out of order. But such an error does not diminish the significance nor the logic of the employed strategies, nor alter the importance of their various outcomes. For as a remarkably complete document of insight into the workings of Ted's self-reliant mind, the worksheet warrants such an attempt and inclusion here.
6. See Table II for a schematic representation of other models' schema of the life course, beyond those cited in the text, and how they bear on Mr. Barrett's history.

REFERENCES

Buhler, C.
1935 The curve of life as studied in biographies. *Journal of Applied Psychology, 19*: 405–409.
Cain, L. D., Jr.
1964 Life course and social structure. In Fairs, R. E. L. (ed.), *Handbook of modern sociology* (pp. 272–309). New York: Rand McNally.
Edgerton, R. B.
1967 *The cloak of competence: Stigma in the lives of the mentally retarded*. Los Angeles: University of California Press.
Erikson, E.
1959 *Identity and the life cycle*: Selected Papers. *Psychological Issues 1*. New York: International Universities Press.
Hart, C. W. M.
1954 The sons of Turimpi. *American Anthropologist, 56*: 242–261.
Jung, C. G.
1931 *Psychology of the unconscious. A study of the transformations and symbolisms of the libido*. New York: Dodd, Mead and Company, c. 1916.
Langness, L. L.
1982 *Mental retardation as an anthropological problem*. Wenner-Gren Foundation Working Papers in Anthropology.
Levinson *et al.*
1974 The psychosocial development of men in early adulthood and in the mid-life transition. In Ricks, D. F. *et al.* (eds.), *Life history research in psychopathology*, (Vol. 3). Minneapolis: University of Minnesota Press.
Linden, M. E. and Dourtney, D.
1953 The human life cycle and its interruptions. *American Journal of Psychiatry, 109*: 906–915.
Miller, D. C. and Form, L. W.
1951 *Industrial sociology: An introduction to the sociology of work relations*. New York: Harper and Row.

HAROLD G. LEVINE AND L. L. LANGNESS

CONCLUSIONS: THEMES IN AN ANTHROPOLOGY OF
MILD MENTAL RETARDATION

The argument for an anthropological study of mental retardation is, now, an old but still valid one. If there is one firm conclusion to be made over the last decade and one-half of research on this handicapping condition, it is that mild mental retardation is as much or more a social and cultural phenomenon as it is a medical-genetic or cognitive-psychological one. In support of this, different researchers have pointed to the instability of definitions of retardation over the years and how definitional changes have directly affected the absolute number of individuals in the population regarded as "retarded". They have demonstrated how each new immigrant group has been "found" to have a disproportionate number of retarded members and how this proportion suspiciously changes as even newer immigrant groups replace the old (Kamin, 1974). Other researchers have shown how purportedly retarded persons sometimes blend in with the general population once they are out of school (MacMillan, 1977); and how, at least in recent times, the school system "conspires" to label and place retarded and other developmentally delayed children in special classes in order to fill quotas and guarantee governmental funding (Mehan et al., 1981; Mehan, 1983; 1984). Finally, although so-called labeling theory has been subject to much criticism and emendation since it was first proposed (Guskin, 1978; Rowitz, 1981; Sagarin, 1975), it is clear that there are important consequences of being labeled retarded, either to the self esteem and subsequent performance of individuals so labeled and/or to the expectations of parents, teachers, peers, and others who surround the labeled individual. The definition of retardation, then, and some of the consequences of being thus labeled are concomitants of social life.

As a sociocultural phenomenon, investigators have already learned a number of important lessons about retardation in general, and the daily lives of retarded persons, in particular. Through the pioneering ethnographic work of Robert Edgerton (1967; Edgerton and Bercovici, 1976; Edgerton, Bollinger and Herr, 1984) and others, as well as life history and autobiographical accounts of and by retarded individuals, we have finally begun to appreciate that the viewpoints of retarded persons themselves must be included in any comprehensive study of retardation. It is only through their voices, and the careful examination of what they say and do in everyday life that we can fully interpret their behavior independently of the label of retardation. That is, we can thereby assess and interpret the effects of settings and significant others on behavior, as well as the understandings and rationalizations which labeled individuals themselves use to explain their own lives. By doing so, we avoid the danger of accounting for behavior in terms of an oversimplified linear

191

L. L. Langness and H. G. Levine (eds.), Culture and Retardation, 191—206.
© 1986 by D. Reidel Publishing Company.

relationship between some ill-defined (and ever-changing) state of retardation as cause and "retarded" behavior as effect. Rather, as with the study of
any other population, we can examine the behavior and beliefs of these
individuals for what they are: as coping strategies, as adaptive mechanisms in
complex situational settings, as cultural solutions to everyday demands, as
learned behavior that "looks" retarded, or perhaps, as behavior which is
ultimately explicable only by recourse to some inherent cognitive or medical
deficiency.

Detailed observations of the lives of retarded persons have reinforced the
already well-supported, but still often overlooked, conclusion that, whatever
else it may be, retarded behavior is not a unitary phenomenon nor do
retarded persons constitute a homogeneous population. The case studies and
observational records which are available, including the papers in the present
volume, attest to the wide diversity of life options exercised, familial pressures and other social constraints activated, and innate skills and learned
competencies realized. Case studies of individuals also force us to acknowledge their *competencies*, sometimes quite hidden from public view, and the
existence of which further strains the credibility of arguments purporting to
define or explain *the* nature of retardation. Clearly, even at a superficial level,
the matter of what retardation "is", and how it manifests itself in everyday
life, are complex, multi-faceted questions.

The fact that it is diversity — behavioral, cognitive, social, and otherwise
— which best seems to characterize the lives of these handicapped individuals presents a peculiar problem for an anthropology of retardation. It
calls into question the applicability of the key explanatory concept of
anthropology — the notion of culture. Certainly, in the most traditional and
common usage, the culture concept would seem inappropriate when applied
to the handicapped. Culture is most commonly conceived of as a property of
groups — those extra-genetically transmitted meanings and ways of understanding that are part of a tradition of learned and shared, if largely
subconscious, designs for living. But the mentally handicapped tend to lead
marginal existences, do not reside contiguously nor even necessarily interface
with one another, do not consciously share any common identity nor a wish
to do so, and cannot possibly share specific sets of knowledge and rules for
action by which they can be identified.

If not in the most traditional sense, then, how does it make sense to apply
the culture concept to the retarded? Following Edward Sapir, we would
argue that "the true locus of culture is in the individual" (1917). And,
following A. Irving Hallowell, we would further argue that to be human at all
is to possess a distinctively cultural mode of existence (1963). As Clifford
Geertz has put it:

. . . there is no such thing as a human nature independent of culture. Men without culture
would not be the clever savages of Golding's *Lord of the Flies* thrown back upon the cruel

wisdom of their animal instincts; nor would they be the nature's noblemen of Enlightenment primitivism or even, as classical anthropological theory would imply, intrinsically talented apes who had somehow failed to find themselves. They would be unworkable monstrosities with very few useful instincts, fewer recognizable sentiments, and no intellect: mental basket cases. As our central nervous system — and most particularly its crowning curse and glory, the neocortex — grew up in great part in interaction with culture, it is incapable of directing our behavior or organizing our experience without the guidance provided by systems of significant symbols. What happened to us in the Ice Age is that we were obliged to abandon the regularity and precision of detailed genetic control over our conduct for the flexibility and adaptability of a more generalized, though of course no less real, genetic control over it. To supply the additional information necessary to be able to act, we were forced, in turn, to rely more and more heavily on cultural sources — the accumulated fund of significant symbols. Such symbols are thus not mere expressions, instrumentalities, or correlates of our biological, psychological, and social existence; they are prerequisites of it. Without men, no culture, certainly; but equally, and more significantly, without culture, no men.

We are, in sum, incomplete or unfinished animals who complete or finish ourselves through culture — and not through culture in general but through highly particular forms of it: Dobuan and Javanese, Hopi and Italian, upper-class and lower-class, academic and commercial. Man's great capacity for learning, his plasticity, has often been remarked, but what is even more critical is his extreme dependence upon a certain sort of learning: the attainment of concepts, the apprehension and application of specific systems of symbolic meaning. Beavers build dams, birds build nests, bees locate food, baboons organize social groups, and mice mate on the basis of forms of learning that rest predominantly on the instructions encoded in their genes and evoked by appropriate patterns of external stimuli: physical keys inserted into organic locks. But men build dams or shelters, locate food, organize their social groups, or find sexual partners under the guidance of instructions encoded in flow charts and blueprints, hunting lore, moral systems, and aesthetic judgments: conceptual structures molding formless talents.

We live, as one writer has neatly put it, in an 'information gap'. Between what our body tells us and what we have to know in order to function, there is a vacuum we must fill ourselves, and we fill it with information (or misinformation) provided by our culture. The boundary between what is innately controlled and what is culturally controlled in human behavior is an ill-defined and wavering one (Geertz, 1965: 112—113).

There can be little doubt that retarded individuals are not also cultural animals like the rest of us. What is at issue, for the anthropologist, is whether mentally handicapped persons master significant symbols in the same way other people do and whether their storehouses of symbols approximate not only each others' but those of non-handicapped individuals as well.

We believe that the answer to these basic questions can be found, at least in part, through an analysis of the kinds of life history materials presented in this volume and in the results of other observational and ethnographic research with retarded individuals. To anticipate our argument, we believe that the culture of retardation, so to speak, can be conceptualized best as a by-product of the widespread *denial* of information about everday life to persons perceived as handicapped. This denial, in turn, has two key components: (1) the *processes* by which certain individuals come to be uninformed of the practical and conceptual knowledge necessary for competence in everyday affairs (and the nature of just what that knowledge is), and (2) the intra- and inter-personal consequences for retarded persons of this lack of information when confronting the everyday world. These components, then, resolve themselves into two traditional anthropological concerns: socialization practices (and the continuing enculturation of adults), and the effects of knowledge and belief systems on individual behavior.

Although we do not yet have a body of research material substantial enough to permit a full discussion of how everyday knowledge becomes unavailable to segments of the population, it is possible to outline some of the general themes which seem to characterize the lives of retarded persons. We organize these themes in terms of the two key components discussed above, and use the life histories presented in this volume and other published ethnographic materials to illustrate them.

I

While researchers are increasingly coming to see the need to investigate the early home experiences of retarded children, particularly the frequency, content, and style of parent-child interactions, and their impact on subsequent cognitive and social development (see Stoneman and Brody, 1982), it is quite clear from life history studies that the *cultural* content and experiences of these children tend to be restricted from an early age. This occurs in a number of different ways, as the data in this volume demonstrate. Overprotective parents do not allow their retarded children to play and develop in the same way as other children. John Millon, for example, vividly remembers going on hikes with his mother, and while the other chidren ran off to investigate something mysterious in the brush, he was held back by his mother lest he be hurt. Restrictions also occur on the child's playmates. John Millon's friends had been picked by his mother because "they were all ones who couldn't do very much, who had something wrong with them" (p. 116). Penny Davis found that, while her mother denied that anything was wrong with Penny's development, other mothers did not. Thus Penny was shunned by her peers, and her opportunities to play even with younger children, while occasionally permitted, were also restricted. We know that Ted Barrett's father abandoned his family when Ted was a child and that the latter's early life was characterized by familial discord, transience, and rejection. Larry B., too, was rejected as a child and adolescent by both parents and a special girlfriend. His feelings of rejection, so painfully expressed in the song lyrics he now writes, seem to reappear forever in his daily life. In spite of the special training he has received for independent living he fails to understand the nuances of tipping and other social conventions appropriate in public places.

The socialized isolation which we see in many retarded children also seems to follow them into adulthood. Kaufman, for example, tells us that her daughter Colette and Colette's retarded friends shared "the realization that potential friendships are limited to marginal members of society". Colette also often revealed that she "knew her place", that somehow she was offensive to nonretarded family members and others and could impose on their lives only with great caution. John Hamlin found himself excluded from certain social activities such as an evening of bar-hopping and dancing. John's insecurity over his social skills, his frequent exclusion from social events, led him to voluntarily exclude himself from such gatherings. In other examples Koegel shows us how Penny Davis came to be rejected by her family, and Whittemore makes painfully clear the isolation and difficulties of Ted Barrett's life.

Because of this isolation and treatment it is not surprising that retarded adults have gaps in their experience and are aware of how differently they have been treated. Thus, we are only mildly surprised to find that Larry B. remains ignorant of the fact that prostitutes will not accept checks or that John Hamlin is shocked to discover men showering in the nude in a communal locker room, and that, in yet another context, he is uncomfortable with unfamiliar menus. We also begin to suspect that John Hamlin is unhappily aware that the behaviors so visible among the male adults in his family — the smoking, drinking, bar-hopping — are denied him but not his brother. Larry B. comments on the different ways he and his sister were raised by their parents, and now Larry finds himself making further invidious comparisons with others with negative consequences for himself and his self image. Colette constantly compares her monotonous xeroxing job with the more varied responsibilities enjoyed by her fellow employees and is depressed by the contrast. Colette also suffers at the contrast between her own limited and shabby material possessions and the more glittering goods in her parent's home. Ted Barrett is well aware of others' recognition of his limitations and entertains the paranoid delusion of being constantly watched.

Not only do isolation and the resulting gaps in knowledge stifle everyday learning and limit everyday competence for those labeled retarded, but also the fact that nonretarded persons assume them to be universally incompetent is further limiting. As several of the authors in this volume have made clear, incompetency in one life domain seems to have inevitable "spill-over" effects into others. John Hamlin, for example, is infantilized to the point that his father refuses to let him slice a cold roast. John Millon, Edgerton informs us, is regarded by his caretakers as emotionally immature and unable to do simple self-maintenance chores. Yet John is quite able to speak out on what he perceives to be the injustices of the caretaking system. He is embittered that workshop personnel maintain that they present real jobs intended for adults, but then proceed to treat the retarded workers as children. Millon points out that "they never have normal peoples work on the same level as these [retarded] people" (p. 120). As to family care homes, John is similarly resentful: "They [the residents] aren't given any type of freedom. There's always someone to keep an eye on them" (p. 121). Kaufman, as another example, notes that Colette's "view of the world was colored by repeated

experiences which indicated to her that she was incompetent" (p. 38). Her
work supervisors thought her incapable of handling the more complicated,
and better-paying positions, and her parents thought her incompetent to own
a car, to manage her finances, and to undertake motherhood.

The case of Colette's "incompetence" with regard to money management
also raises an interesting point about the relationship of incompetence to
individual motivation. We know from her mother's account that Colette felt
that she needed to buy a large number of items and was unable to do so
because of a lack of money. Colette's mother responded, almost predictably,
with the assertion that the real problem might not lie in how much money
Colette had, but in how she managed what she did have. At this point in
their discussion Colette defends herself and makes it clear that, whether
or not she knows how to manage her funds, her preferences lie elsewhere.
Rather than stay home, worry, and manage her money to pay the rent and
buy other necessities, she would rather enjoy herself by going out and
spending money. Thus, Colette is placed in a kind of double-bind. If she does
as others wish, she has her rent paid but is bored; but if she does as she
wishes, she will (she claims) enjoy life but have to face others' assumption of
her incompetency. Colette, like other retarded persons, continually redis-
covers that her actions are open to the scrutiny of others. It is a scrutiny,
moreover, which focuses neither on the meaning of the action nor its value to
the individual, but its testimony to the intellectual competence and responsibility of the actor.

The assumed incompetency and the infantilization of retarded persons
seems to extend in one further direction. In none of the accounts presented
here and elsewhere in the literature do we find much parental or service
delivery system concern or support for the emotional states of retarded
persons. Yet the enforced isolation to which retarded persons are subject
surely extends to life events which often carry deep emotional consequences.
Indeed, one of the themes that most clearly emerges from life histories is
that retarded persons, just as others, are subject, periodically, to severe psychological stress. It may be that their general inability to find a sympathetic
ear and, perhaps, a lack of experience in how to grapple with stress may
place them under even greater emotional duress than would otherwise be the
case. Whatever, they often seem to suffer in virtual silence. Larry B., for
example, constantly dwells on his lack of female companionship which he
attributes to his lack of worldliness. He ruminates over a former girlfriend
who jilted him, and expresses this frustration in violent fantasies designed to
harm her. Also we learn that, at age 15, Larry had to face the drowning of
his girlfriend who, in retrospect at least, he was to marry when they both
turned 18. We learn that Penny Davis has affective needs which she seems to
satisfy with apparently superficial and transitory affairs with men. Ted
Barrett worries over his advancing age and seems shaken by his perception
of his own irreversible loss of sexual potency.

As social and emotional isolates, retarded individuals lead, almost without exception in the accounts here, marginal lives. They are typically not part of the mainstream and, with their powerlessness and lack of everyday experience, seem sadly at its mercy. Indeed, it is common to find that their lives are often studied by social scientists using theories derived for other marginal or deviant individuals (see, e.g., Biklen, 1977; Edgerton, 1967; Farber, 1968). Whatever their marginal status may be, however, it is important to note that it is produced by a highly differentiated set of socialization practices which tend to deny retarded persons familiarity with, and opportunities to learn through, normal experience.

The papers in this volume help to make clear how retarded persons are subtly (or even blatantly) socialized for incompetence. This implies a degree of universality in the childrearing practices of the parents of retarded children. Thus, while it is true that the retarded do not share a common culture, they may likely share similar deficits in enculturative experiences. These may exacerbate whatever problems the retarded may have initially been thought to have, and may result in channeling them into the psychological and actual physical margins of society's mainstream. In support of these propositions we observe that parents seem to place more restrictions on their retarded children and, according to some of the accounts offered here, are genuinely confused about what their children's learning problems and expected abilities may be. We note also that peer learning is limited, and that retarded children often must reply on even younger children as playmates. Under these circumstances they encounter age inappropriate tasks. As Korbin points out, they become increasingly out of the synchronization with cultural expectations. The mature development of even simple everyday heuristics may be denied to them because of their abbreviated interactions with parents and same-age peers, and because of their impoverished real-world experience base. In effect they are denied the social and interactional milieus within which everyday problems are embedded and solution strategies first expressed (cf. Cole and Griffin, 1983; Levine and Langness, 1985; Vygotsky, 1978). One practical consequence of this is that many retarded persons never develop the sequences of trying, failing, and learning from mistakes, nor do they develop specific problem-solving strategies. While supporting data for these points remain inconclusive at present, there is some comparative evidence that retarded children who are forced to be more independent of their families or who are included in everyday transactions by their parents later develop into the most flexible, competent adult everyday problem solvers (see Levine and Langness, 1985).

Many of the problems which plague the normal socialization of retarded children continue into their adulthood as well. Full enculturation rarely occurs because, still isolated, the friends of retarded persons are likely to be other marginal members of society. Cumulative inexperience constantly makes them seem out of place and seems to promote self-doubt and uncertainty. Perhaps most importantly, retarded adults, as several authors have observed here, do not have available to them the traditional markers which indicate success in the world or which signify the appropriate transitions through life stages. In particular, age itself has no value, either as a guarantor of certain abilities or as a claim for certain prerogatives in the world at large.

With little ability to judge or measure their lives against some societal standard, and with others shunning them in one form or another, retarded adults remain "frozen" in time, not children but never really accepted as adults. Denied the standard accoutrements of enhanced status and age, they have nothing to expect as they mature. Inevitably there is always something missing from their lives, and if their lives in some way are shaped by personal passages or critical incidents (see Whittemore, Langness and Koegel, this volume) these remain elusive. We lack a developmental theory for handicapped individuals.

Interestingly, the socialization practices we use for handicapped individuals are themselves part of a distinctive cultural tradition which sees the developmentally delayed as children, and, as such, with little need to learn or understand many of the ordinary facts of everyday life. Indeed, we believe it is better for them *not* to learn certain things. And, as this same cultural tradition places a great value on efficiency and speed, it is easier to tie their shoes for them than wait for them to do it themselves, easier to deliver them to the workshop than teach them to use the bus, and in general easier to deny them experience than to deal with their presumed or potential failures. Thus the socialization of the retarded, whatever its various motives, appears almost as a cultural conspiracy which produces an effect quite the opposite of that intended. The lack of opportunity and experience denies specific knowledge of many everyday affairs which is essential for normal life. Of equal importance, the knowledge and thinking processes learned from engaging in everyday events and problems is also denied.

II

Improper socialization, isolation, and the lack of developmental milestones for retarded persons appear to have a variety of additional consequences for their lives. While reading the accounts presented here, we are struck by the loneliness some of these people endure and the self-reliance they develop to cope with their many and varied social and emotional problems. However, we are also struck by the fact that, at times, they wish to be left alone or that there are certain areas of their lives where they fight for privacy. Thus, Colette's relationship with her lover Edgar and her financial troubles were disallowed topics of conversation between Colette and her mother. It is precisely in these areas that Colette needs to prove her competence without either her mother's interference or implied criticism. Penny Davis, as another example, resents the intrusion of the various social workers sent to help her and resists being made to conform to the middle-class way of life deemed suitable for her by the service delivery system. In spite of his loneliness, Larry B. rejects any association with other retarded persons, and Ted Barrett refuses to move into subsidized housing or to his sister's horse farm in the California high desert, both places where his standard of living (but also his boredom) would rise substantially.

Fundamental questions about the self also seem to be a consequence of years of questionable socialization, mistaken diagnosis, and bewildered parents. The life histories in this volume demonstrate that one of the tragedies of mental retardation is its impact on the lives of those so labeled. Larry B., for example, in his confusion about what mental retardation is, and whether he believes the term is self-descriptive, variously links it with his violent fantasies toward his former girlfriend, "brain damage", mental illness (or "craziness"), his loneliness, and adult immaturity. At one point he even wonders whether his sister could have placed a spell on him as she once threatened to do. In general, he is described as tense and worried a great deal of the time, in particular whether others may be able to look at him and determine that he is retarded. Not surprisingly, Larry also manufactures rationalizations to account for his behavior, and, at the same time, to liken it to that of others. He tells his interviewer:

> Do you remember I told you I wasn't exactly mature for my age? I think I was being hard on myself when I said I was emotionally immature because I think everyone is emotional to a certain degree. I think everyone has some craziness in them. I think everyone is immature up to a certain degree and I even think everyone has some child[ish]ness in them. I even think everyone has a certain amount of retardation in them. I even think that people have a little hoodishness in them. They get a little smart alecky or sneaky or slightly delinquent at times . . . (p. 76).

For John Millon being retarded means being "irrational, doing weird things with no cause behind it" (p. 119), but John is also confused about mental testing and the meaning of I.Q. scores. John has apparently become accustomed to his incompetent self-image, but after being de-labeled and expected to be competent he makes mistakes or worries that he will do so. For Ted Barrett, too, one of his central concerns in life is his competence, and he worries about his ability at "figuring even confusing things out" (p. 158). In Ted's mind not only are mental retardation and incompetence probably linked, but they are marked by his inability to read and write. Even so, and in spite of Ted's partial recognition of his own limitations, we learn from Whittemore that Ted probably has always been confused by the retardation label (p. 165). Finally, in the life histories of Ed Murphy and Pattie Burt as presented by Bogdan and Taylor (1982), we are told that their stories

> . . . are testimonials to the ability of human beings to survive the systematic and brutal attack on the self, [but that] they also reveal that such attacks leave scars, even on the strongest of the

subjected. Pat and Ed's reflections on the present reveal self-concepts that have been shaken. While they do not define their 'selves' as retarded, there are traces of gnawing doubts about themselves in their thoughts. (1982: 219)

Further, Pat acknowledges feeling "abnormal" (Bogdan and Taylor, 1982: 219).

Such self-doubts for retarded adults, coupled with their marginal status and general lack of success in the world, seem to result in serious losses of self-esteem, an observation first significantly addressed by Edgerton in *The Cloak of Competence*. For the individuals studied here, their self-esteem seems shaken by the negative attitudes held by others, by the inferior ways in which they see themselves being treated by their parents when compared with nonretarded siblings, and by the daily adversities they face in having their social, financial, and emotional needs met.

The constant threats to self-esteem, the stigma of being labeled retarded, the denial by others of crucial information about everyday matters, and the never-ending social isolation of retarded adults would seem to be crippling for the day-to-day functioning of anyone. For retarded persons one might expect passivity and dependency upon others. We would particularly expect to discover this accommodation strategy for those persons who have been insitutionalized, since passivity in the face of institutional demands and time schedules would be highly adaptive. We also find merit in the argument (Edgerton, this volume) that retarded persons and their service system residential caretakers participate in a delicate, but nevertheless mutual and effective, collusion which keeps the retarded person compliant, incompetent, and, hence, retarded. In the trade-off between caretaker and retarded client, the former gains a livelihood and smooth-running residential operation and the latter a home and a predictable and undemanding environment.

The classic response of retarded persons to this set of social conditions has been successfully portrayed by Edgerton (1967). In his study of 48 formerly institutionalized mildly retarded adults, Edgerton found three key ingredients in their efforts to cope with the stigma of being labeled as retarded and the attendant threats to self-esteem. The first two of these were denial and passing. All of the members of his study sample denied that they were retarded and found other explanations for their incarceration in an institution for mentally retarded people. Most typically they saw their *release* from the institution as confirmation of their belief that they never belonged there in the first place. Once out of the institution they then developed a "cover" story to explain, but also to conceal, their institutional history.

Release from the institution also brought other problems to the retarded adults of Edgerton's study. The real problems of everyday life had to be solved, not only to survive and avoid re-incarceration, but also to avoid the appearance of seeming retarded. The most troublesome of these problems were making a living, finding a mate, managing material possessions, and maintaining competence in interpersonal relations. In each of these the "trick" to passing was achieved in somewhat different ways. As to the first two, merely finding and holding a job and finding a mate, preferably a marriage partner, were in themselves status enhancing and came to symbolize freedom from institutional restraints. These ex-patients also put great energy into accumulating possessions. They often frequented junk shops to purchase personal souvenirs which they used to conceal the lack of a real history with the everyday world. They purchased books and magazines which they could not, or would not, read, but displayed prominently in their homes as they had seen nonretarded persons do. They collected real and bogus letters so as to seem surrounded by mail. And for those who could manage it, they looked for cars, even if they did not run, to present "the ultimate symbol of success" (Edgerton, 1967: 160) to the outside world.

Finally, in the arena of interpersonal skills the retarded adults studies by Edgerton quite easily generated covering strategies to solve the dilemmas at hand when they were without the specific skills to solve a given task. Examples include functionally illiterate individuals who claimed they had forgotton their glasses when called upon to read; persons unable to tell time deliberately wearing a broken watch so that others could legitimately be asked for the time; persons with poor counting and arithmetic skills presenting large denomination bills at supermarket check-out stands so that the clerk had to do the necessary calculations prior to dispensing any change; and so on.

The third ingredient in Edgerton's account of how ex-patients coped with life's demands was for them to enlist the aid of well-meaning benefactors. Almost all of the 48 persons in Edgerton's study had connected with such helpers. These benefactors variously included spouses, landladies, employers, social workers, neighbors, and relatives. They not only helped the retarded person with the manifold exigencies of everyday life, but through a kind and tacit collusion aided in denial and passing.

Edgerton's pioneering account does not speak in detail about the positive features of his subject population. From the evidence presented in this volume it seems that there are additional features which figure into how retarded adults cope with everday demands and some deviation from the situation as presented by Edgerton. As to the latter, while all the subjects of these studies on whom we have information generally deny their retardation, they are not always able to do so. Some subjects, when confronted about it, agree that it is self-descriptive. More importantly, none of the persons discussed here seem particularly concerned with finding a mentor-benefactor. In several cases, e.g., Colette, Penny Davis, Ted Barrett, they actively rejected help when it would not come in an acceptable form. Ted Barrett, moreover, himself became a benefactor to his friend Valerie and her son Richard.

With the exception of John Hamlin who seems dependent upon his parents and acknowledges, however unwillingly, their final authority over his life, all the others studied here reveal a remarkable independence in some ways. We see Colette's resentment toward her mother and her steadfastness in denying her family's unwanted intrusion into the secret places of her life. We hear Larry B.'s anger toward the world, toward board and care facilities in particular, and his eventual success in obtaining a job and moving into an apartment by himself. Much of the same bitterness toward "the system" we find in John Millon's words. Penny Davis remains incorrigible and resourceful to the end. Not willing to accept the middle-class values and morals which various social workers would have her adopt, she seizes new opportunities to meet new people, especially men, with whom she can bond. She seems little bothered by the resulting insecurity and constant upheaval in her life. Ted Barrett is a survivor, someone whose independence and resourcefulness allow him to deal with the complexities and dangers of living in the inner city. Tim Anthony overcomes a childhood of poverty and abuse, rises above his family and early trauma to make an unusually successful attempt at a "normal" life.

The resourcefulness of these individuals shows up in other ways. Colette and Edgar rent a car when they are unable to purchase one, and Colette finds a way of having the Department of Rehabilitation underwrite her driver training. John Hamlin works in a factory, has a job with responsibility, and negotiates four hours of bus travel with numerous transfers to get to and from work. Penny Davis is resourceful enough to arrive in Los Angeles from New York without a place to stay and to find shelter with a stranger in his motel room. Ted Barrett negotiates the inner city with unusual but successful finesse. Although "handicapped", these are in many ways resourceful people. They make do with what they have. While they do not solve their problems in what might always be seen as culturally appropriate ways, they do often solve them.

In spite of the experiential limitations stemming from an often haphazard socialization process, these persons seem to learn how to survive even with limited information about how the world works. We find striking independence and resourcefulness as they negotiate the trials and pitfalls of everyday life. The occasional use of benefactors who offer some external competence and familiarity with problematic tasks, of "covering" or "meta" strategies to deal with inability or unfamiliarity, and of largely private islands of competency where skills and resourcefulness may be tried are all ways of learning to cope but without actually learning any of the subtleties by which the world is organized. This form of learning may be highly adaptive for the retarded person as he or she goes about negotiating everyday life; but paradoxically, its adaptiveness continues to inhibit the reversal to any basic deficits in skill learning or any gaps in everyday knowledge which their socialization may have forced upon them. Being "retarded" in this culture is thus a curious mix of competence and incompetence, of using one's skills and resourcefulness to assess everyday demands and needs and then to find ways around fundamental gaps in knowledge. Even with this resourcefulness, however, available evidence indicates that the intro- and interpersonal consequences of being labeled retarded, particularly in terms of threats to self-esteem, are potentially enormous. It is yet another way in which handicapping conditions for this population may be characterized.

To ignore the historical and socio-cultural contexts within which retardation occurs is to render the complexity of retardation into an oversimplified "condition" — something one has or does not have that may be referenced to some underlying medical or cognitive deficiency. Certainly the history of studies on retardation seem so directed; find the quick diagnosis, the seeming cause, the inevitable consequence, and one has "explained" retardation. If we start with the premise that retarded persons are different, scientific concern will inevitably be directed toward finding *the* nature of the difference. In this last section we wish to explore a research agenda which starts with a different premise. What if retarded persons are, if not quite the same as the rest of us, not *quite* so different? What if, in other words, we acknowledge their common humanity but also their marginality? What more will this tell us about retardation itself and, equally important to the social scientist, the nature of *not* being retarded?

Although the life histories presented here, and our summary discussion of them, cannot be considered the final proof, traditional anthropological concerns with socialization, with knowledge systems, and with everyday thought and problem solving seem highly appropriate to any discussion of mental retardation. Certainly, more ethnographic work of this sort with this population is in order since relatively so little is known about marginality, let alone the large variety of life experiences and adaptations made by mentally handicapped individuals. Anthropological interest in this population must be seen as highly consistent with the studies of other segments, whether marginal or not, of American society.

Studies of subgroups within the United States, while certainly valuable in their own right, offer another advantage also consonant with the logic of anthropological investigation. Anthropologists have always gone off to the bush somewhere, not only to generate a genuinely meaningful study of the human condition, but also to gain perspectives on their own society. The logic has been one of casting off one's cultural blinders by examining the form and function of others' cultural practices. Equally important, part of the anthropological "logic of inquiry" is the study of antitheses, certainly *between* cultures but *within* given cultural traditions as well. Thus, one can learn something of normalcy by the study of deviance (e.g., Edgerton, 1976) or the nature of sanity by examining *in*sanity (e.g., Wilson, 1974). Cultural antitheses can be thought of, in fact, as a kind of imperfect natural laboratory wherein controlled comparison is a feasible goal. Under these conditions the manifold practices and beliefs which the word "culture" glosses can be

204 H. G. LEVINE AND L. L. LANGNESS

roughly equated so that the institution or set of practices of particular concern can be isolated for study. In principle, the distinguishing features which set, say, a deviant career or a psychiatric episode in motion for one set of individuals can be separately charted from the circumstances which lead others in the same culture down other paths without the confounding effect of having been born in radically different cultures.

Given value in the study of antitheses as a classic anthropological strategy, what can be learned about the study of the lives of mentally retarded individuals? The variety of scientifically appropriate answers to this question seems clear. Labeling phenomena, stigma, coping and adaptation, stress and self-esteem, and the nature of competence are clear choices. Another choice, on a larger scale, has been explored by Turner (1982) in his account of a sheltered workshop. Turner argues for looking at the workshop as a kind of microcosm of the larger society where tensions between "instrumentality" (task requirements, authority structure, rules, production demands) and "expressiveness" (social support, sense of belonging, friendship, sense of self-worth) are played out as in any larger human community. Turner provocatively argues that the "focal concerns" of workshop members "are not 'mentally retarded concerns': they are the concerns of all people" (1982: 42).

From our point of view there is a further, critically important avenue of inquiry which is made possible by the ethnographic investigation of retarded persons. Certainly, one of the abiding values of American society is intelligence, particularly the kind manifested in intelligence tests, formal schooling, and laboratory tasks developed to study cognition. Interestingly, we also seem to recognize a "second" intelligence, not as prized as the first, perhaps, but valued in many ways as well. We speak of "native intelligence", of "commonsense", of "hard-won experience". We speak of individuals as having learned from the "college of hard-knocks" or as having "learned by doing". The culture seems to recognize two distinct kinds of intelligence, formal and everyday. To date, we have very few studies of the latter and, as one consequence, no way of meshing what we know about thinking under formal conditions whith that exhibited during everyday circumstances (Levine, Zetlin and Langness, 1980). Just how to go about studying thinking in its everyday context is also not clear since generally accepted guidelines for doing so have not been forthcoming. We guess that one reason for this lack is that everyday thought is not a significant issue for the academic community where formal thinking is the *sine qua non* of intelligence. Another reason is likely to be that everyday thinking, because of its pervasiveness and "familiarity", tends to be taken for granted. It becomes, in a way, invisible.

One research strategy for making the invisible visible is to study the phenomenon in a place where it is visible. Errors in thinking, both formal and everyday thought, is a common element of standard definitions of retardation. Retarded persons are just those persons who are not very "smart", for whom thought of all kinds is *the* problematic of their lives.

Therefore, by the logic of antitheses, we should be able to learn something about thinking by examining the lives of persons who are "unable" to think. However, the emphasis here is not in further uncovering and explaining cognitive deficiencies, but rather, in finding the demands of various settings and the nature of thinking which is required in these settings. To this end we must follow retarded persons into supermarkets (Levine and Langness, 1985), buses, banks, fast-food restaurants, job sites, bowling alleys, and the like. We must look for errors in logic, site and personnel demands, inter-action about cognition, background experience and its consequences for current performance, and other clues which may help us understand how much of what we think is "internal" and how much is keyed to the social and interactional milieus of which thinking is a part.

The suggestions we have put forth here are not intended to exhaust a research agenda focused on retardation. Indeed, as anthropologists we particularly need to continue the limited amount of cross-cultural research which has been done. The goal, here, must be additional data relevant to cross-cultural socialization practices, labeling practices, and life experience. Extensive research in these areas may also enable us to sort out how much of what we call mental retardation is ultimately contextual or cultural and how much is connected with some set of bottomline conditions of the human mind. It is to this end that anthropological research in mental retardation has its greatest contribution to make.

ACKNOWLEDGEMENT

The authors wish to thank R. B. Edgerton and J. R. Newbrough for their thoughtful reviews of the manuscript.

REFERENCES

Biklen, D.
   1977 Myths, mistreatment, and pitfalls: Mental retardation and criminal justice. *Mental Retardation, 15*: 51—57.
Bogdan, R. and Taylor, S. J.
   1982 *Inside out: Two first person accounts of what it means to be labled 'mentally retarded'*. Toronto: University of Toronto Press.
Cole, M. and Griffin, P.
   1983 A socio-historical approach to remediation. *The Quarterly Newsletter of the Laboratory of Comparative Human Cognition, 5*: 69—74.
Edgerton, R. B.
   1967 *The Cloak of competence; Stigma in the lives of the mentally retarded*. Berkeley: University of California Press.
Edgerton, R. B.
   1976 *Deviance: A cross-cultural perspective*. Menlo Park, CA: Cummings Publishing.
Edgerton, R. B. and Bercovici, S. M.
   1976 The cloak of comeptence: Years later. *American Journal of Mental Deficiency 80*: 485—497.

Edgerton, R. B., Bollinger, M. and Herr, B.
    1984 The cloak of competence: After two decades. *American Journal of Mental Deficiency, 88*: 345—351.
Farber, B.
    1968 *Mental retardation: Its social context and social consequences.* Boston: Houghton Mifflin Co.
Geertz, C.
    1965 The impact of the concept of culture on the concept of man. *In* J. R. Platt (ed.), *New views of the nature of man,* (pp. 93—118). Chicago: University of Chicago Press.
Guskin, S. L.
    1978 Theoretical and empirical strategies for the study of the labeling of mentally retarded persons. *In* N. R. Ellis (ed.), *International review of research in mental retardation,* Vol. 9 (pp. 127—158). New York: Academic Press.
Hallowell, A. I.
    1963 Personality, culture and society in behavioral evolution. *In* Sigmund Koch (ed.), *Psychology: A study of a science,* Vol. 6 (pp. 429—509). New York: McGraw-Hill.
Kamin, L. J.
    1974 *The science and politics of I.Q.* Potomac, Maryland: Erlbaum.
Levine, H. G., Zetlin, A. G. and Langness, L. L.
    1980 Everyday memory tasks in classrooms for TMR learners. *Quarterly Newsletter of the Laboratory of Comparative Human Cognition, 2*: 1—6.
Levine, H. G. and Langness, L. L.
    1985 Everyday cognition among mildly mentally retarded adults: An ethnographic approach. *American Journal of Mental Deficiency, 90*: 18—26.
MacMillan, D. L.
    1977 *Mental retardation in school and society.* Boston: Little—Brown.
Mehan, H., Meihls, J. L., Hertweck, A. and Crowdes, M. S.
    1981 Identifying handicapped students. *In* S. B. Bacharach (ed.), *Organizational behavior in schools and school districts* (pp. 381—427). New York: Praeger.
Mehan, H.
    1983 The role of language and the language of role in institutional decision making. *Language in Society, 12*: 187—211.
Mehan, H.
    1984 Institutional decision-making. *In* B. Rogoff and J. Lave, (eds.), *Everyday cognition: Its development in social context* (pp. 43—66). Cambridge, MA: Harvard University Press.
Rowitz, L.
    1981 A sociological perspective on labeling in mental retardation. *Mental Retardation, 19*: 47—51.
Sagarin, E.
    1975 *Deviants and deviance: An introduction to the study of disvalued people and behavior.* New York: Praeger.
Sapir, E.
    1917 Do we need a superorganic? *American Anthropologist, 19*: 441—447.
Stoneman, Z. and Brody, G. H.
    1982 Observational research on retarded children, their parents, and their siblings. Paper presented at the Lake Wilderness Conference on the impact of residential evironments on retarded persons and their care providers. Lake Wilderness, Washington.
Vygotsky, L. S.
    1978 *Mind in society.* M. Cole, V. John-Steiner, S. Scribner and E. Souberman (eds.). Cambrige, MA: Harvard University Press.
Wison, P. J.
    1974 *Oscar: An inquiry into the nature of sanity.* New York: Random House.

LIST OF CONTRIBUTORS

Robert B. Edgerton, Ph.D. (Anthropology); Professor, Department of Psychiatry and Biobehavioral Sciences, University of California at Los Angeles, Los Angeles, California.

Linda Hubbard, M.A. (Anthropology); Doctoral Candidate, Department of Anthropology, University of California at Los Angeles, Los Angeles, California.

Sandra Z. Kaufman, M.A. (Education); Research Associate, Department of Psychiatry and Biobehavioral Sciences, University of California at Los Angeles, Los Angeles, California.

Kristina Kennann, Ph.D. (Anthropology); Research Project Manager, Rehabilitation Research and Training Center in Mental Retardation, University of Oregon at Eugene, Eugene, Oregon.

Keith T. Kernan, Ph.D. (Anthropology); Associate Professor, Department of Psychiatry and Biobehavioral Sciences, University of California at Los Angeles, Los Angeles, California.

Paul Koegel, Ph.D. (Anthropology); Associate Director, Mentally Ill Homeless on Skid Row Study, Los Angeles County Department of Mental Health, Los Angeles, California.

Jill E. Korbin, Ph.D. (Anthropology); Assistant Professor, Department of Anthropology, Case Western Reserve University, Cleveland, Ohio; Congressional Fellowship in Child Development for 1985—86.

Lewis L. Langness, Ph.D. (Anthropology); Professor, Department of Psychiatry and Biobehavioral Sciences, University of California at Los Angeles, Los Angeles, California.

Harold G. Levine, Ph.D. (Anthropology); Assistant Professor, Graduate School of Education, University of California at Los Angeles, Los Angeles, California.

Jim L. Turner, Ph.D. (Psychology); Associate Director, Center for Faculty Development, University of California at Long Beach, Long Beach, California.

Robert D. Whittemore, M.A. (Anthropology); Acting Assistant Professor, Reed College, Portland, Oregon.

L. L. Langness and H. G. Levine (eds.), Culture and Retardation, 207.
© 1986 *by D. Reidel Publishing Company.*

INDEX

adaptation 204
  to community living 81–100
  individual 127–155
  social support and 150
adaptive behavior ix, 183–187
adaptive competence 155–189
adaptive mechanisms 191
adaptive strategies 9–12
age 198
age-competence incongruity 20–21, 29–30
aging process 167–168
Aid to the Disabled (ATD) 109–110
alcohol 12–13, 52–58
  see also drinking
antitheses, cultural 203–205
"arc of life," distortion of 13
attribution 101
autobiographies 4–6
automobile driving 41–42, 122
automobile ownership 41–43

Barrett, Theodore V., subject xiii–xiv, 14,
    155–189, 194, 195, 199
  identity 188–189
behavior
  adaptive ix, 183–187
  influences on 194
  retarded 191
benefactors 201
board and care facilities 61, 74–78
brain damage 65, 106, 108
brain-damage etiology 8

caretakers, interest in restriction 123
childhood of retarded persons 19–28, 82–
    83, 85–88, 106–109, 131–132
childrearing, of retarded persons 197
children, equating with xi, 13–14, 30, 50,
    56–61, 194–195
  see also infantilization
communication deficiencies 2, 24–25, 27–28
communication skills 53

community, living in the ix, x, 191
  adaptation to 81–100
  demands of 205
  problems of 200–201
Community Adaptation of Mildly Retarded
    Persons Study 62, 125, 151
Community Context of Normalization Study
    15, 62, 151
companionship 70–73
competence
  adaptive 155–189
  islands of 202
  labeling and 124
  learned 191
  nature of 204
  processes that hinder acquisition of 193–
    194
  socialization and 47, 124
  strategies for 183
  see also incompetence; socialization for
    incompetence
coping 192–204
counting 25–26
covering strategies 200–201
"craziness" 161–165, 168, 189
cultural solutions 191
culture, mental retardation and x, 192–194

delabeling 9–11, 48, 49
  case of 101–126
  effects of 105–106
  reaction to 111–122
delinquency 108
denials of retardation 89–93, 96, 200–201
  processes of 193–194
dependence 200
developmental experience of the retarded
    197–198
developmental interpretation of retardation
    187
developmental milestones and markers 13–
    14, 56

209

DATE DUE			
NO 05 '02			
GAYLORD			PRINTED IN U.S.A.